Paul Barrington Jones

Pearls of Wisdom, Gems of Knowledge for All

Paul Barrington Jones

Pearls of Wisdom, Gems of Knowledge for All

ISBN/EAN: 9783337248505

Printed in Europe, USA, Canada, Australia, Japan

Cover: Foto ©Thomas Meinert / pixelio.de

More available books at **www.hansebooks.com**

PEARLS OF WISDOM,

GEMS OF KNOWLEDGE

FOR ALL.

COMMON SENSE PRESCRIPTIONS AND PRACTICAL INFORMATION.
A SYSTEMATIC TREATMENT IN THE DOMESTIC
PRACTICE OF MEDICINE,

—BY—

PAUL BARRINGTON JONES, M. D.

COPYRIGHT APPLIED FOR.

SOLD BY THE AUTHOR AND HIS AGENTS ONLY.

KANSAS CITY:
Isaac P. Moore, Printer, 12 W. Missouri Ave.
1880.

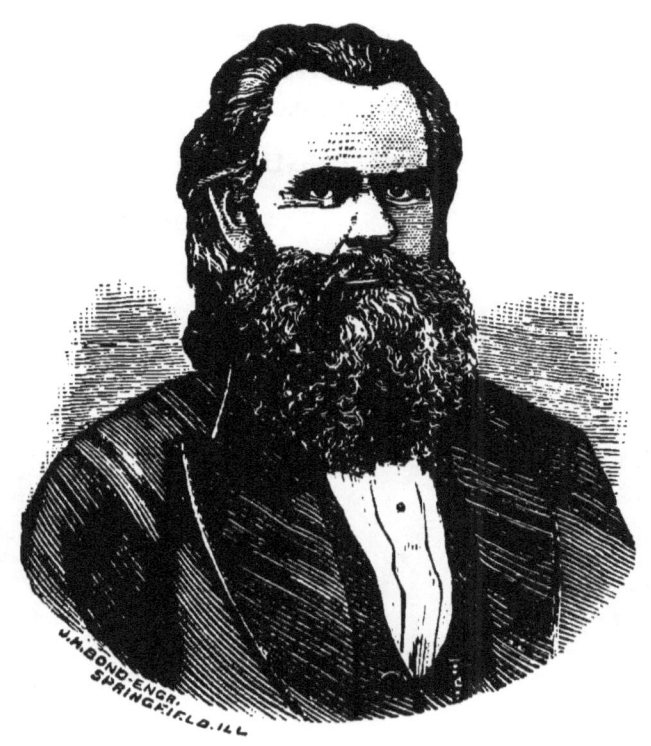

PAUL BARRINGTON JONES, M. D.,
AUTHOR AND PUBLISHER.

THIS LITTLE BOOK
IS DEDICATED
TO MY INESTIMABLE FRIEND,

MR. J. J. HUGHES.

THE AUTHOR.

PREFACE.

The object of placing this little book before the heads of families, and non-professional persons, is to furnish them with a few useful hints and suggestions for those who may be sick as well as to those who have the care of the sick. In the practice of over twenty years, by the bed-side of the sick and misfortunate, we have long since been impressed with the necessity of some kind of a little cheap book which we might place in the hands of every family, which would not only instruct them how to keep well but give them some useful information that would enable them to properly care for the sick, that thousands of lives might be saved from the grave, especially in the case of little children. As the doctor visits from house to house we find many persons thrown into the sick room to care for them, who are exceedingly anxious to know more of their duty. This book is not intended to take the place of a doctor when one is really needed, but more especially to instruct you to do many things that are highly necessary for you to know as well as the doctor, together with much other useful information, such as I know will be highly prized by every household.

THE AUTHOR.

A Good Nurse.

We begin this little book with the above caption and commence to talk plainly of the duties and qualifications of the nurse, for we believe that the cure of the patient depends largely upon the quality and intelligence as well as the adaptation of the nurse; indeed, the great man Valpau once said, "It is the good nurse that saves the sick." Take this view of the matter, the question of her or his duties and qualifications should not be passed over lightly, but should engage our earnest attention.

Some writer has made the statement that "Nurses are like poets and artists—were born, not made." Evidently there are some gifts that are very essential to a good nurse; but we believe that some qualifications may be acquired, and that a little training will often compensate for the lack of natural endowments.

The reason that we have so few good nurses is, because the majority know but little about those things which go to make up what a good nurse should be.

1. *A nurse should be of middle age.* If she is young, she is apt to be thoughtless, wild and heedless; if she or he is old, they may be deaf, or stupid, or in trouble. But a good nurse should be always able to hold herself or himself in subjection, and some old mothers may have all the freshness and acuteness of earlier years. But no matter who the nurse is, she should always wear a cheerful face, no matter how grave the case may be; she should be gentle, kind and obliging; she should always keep calm, not get excited; she must have a pleasant voice, a gentle touch, a light step, and a knowledge of cooking for the sick. Such a person is invaluable.

2. She should be honest—honest with the patient and with the physician.

3. Now, if the patient can have no confidence in the nurse, then the sick-room is no place for such a person; or if the conduct is such as to lead the physician to conclude that his orders have not been

followed, it is certainly a very unfortunate place to occupy; however, no person should employ a physician unless they have confidence in him, after which they should understand his directions; then see to it that you faithfully carry out his orders. Some nurses are very self-opinionated, and they fancy that they know far better than the medical man; and in order to carry out their measures they resort to a species of dishonesty. Such a nurse should be scrupulously avoided, for she ought to know that under the circumstances the patient is made to suffer and perhaps die. A quackish nurse, who gives medicines not ordered by the physician, is an abomination.

4. *A nurse must have sobriety.* Every nurse should be cheerful and pleasant. Some people are always in a constant giggle or titter; the grin of childish levity and thoughtless noise, and roaring laughter, should be avoided: in short, no person should be allowed in the sick room who cannot control themselves. The next quality should be *firmness;* every nurse should be resolute but not rude. She is not expected to yield to the patient every request, unless it comes within the bounds of reason and common sense; everything that is expected to be done she must do cheerfully and kindly, as well as carefully, then after it is done the patient will have confidence in her and praise her for it, and for the exercise of a good judgement.

5. *The next quality is patience.* A very large degree of patience is required, for the reason that sick persons are very often irritable and restless, and sometimes well persons get a touch of it; remember that. Have you not often felt yourself a little ashamed of your own irritability sometimes? I have. Then how would you expect it otherwise with those who are compelled to lie in bed and suffer pain for days, and perhaps weeks, and be deprived of their liberty to even walk about the house? Therefore, it does not matter how sorely tired and worn-out the nurse may be, it does not furnish an excuse for getting out of patience.

She should possess gentleness, in case of a broken limb, painful back, or rheumatism, etc., where it becomes necessary to change the clothing. This requires a good deal of gentleness. The patient should not be handled with an unsteady hand; the holds that secure firmness, strength and gentleness will secure confidence in the invalid and make him feel secure. If you are to do the work, do it with gentleness and not with jerks and knocks, as if you were mad and did not care.

6. *The sixth qualification is cleanliness.* The nurse should not only keep herself clean but she should keep the room clean, neat and sweet. Little filthy things about the room, sticking in the corners, so often spoils the appetite of the patient; never allow the dressings of wounds

or burns to remain in the room; let every vessel be kept empty and clean, ready for use at a moment's warning; then you can let in a little fresh air, by opening a window or door. Remember this must be attended to. Bad air is poisonous. The food not eaten should be taken out of sight; the drinking water should be changed often, as water gathers impurities directly. Be clean in everything you do, and you will be amply rewarded for it.

KINDS OF NURSES.

Some good-hearted people never become good nurses; they seem too awkward and tired, hence they are always overwhelmed in difficulties. They are good-natured creatures, don't mean anything bad, but they can't help it.

Here she comes all loaded down with good things; both hands are full. She goes up stairways, stepping upon the bottom of her dress until she drops a plate or two, or spills the tea, or goes down herself. She manages to get up after a while, and spreads the remainder before the patient. She then cuts the bread and butters it with a knife that has previously been used to cut an onion or spread a mustard plaster, and says, "Now, dear, I will go go back and make some more tea." The patient asks for a drink of water before she goes. She says "yes, dear," and runs off and gets a glass brim full, puts her hand under the patient's head, bends his or her neck, and turns the water down on the outside all over the breast and clothing. Then she wonders why in the world he don't drink better. She lights the lamp, turns the wick up, takes a bit of paper, makes a flash, throws the paper on the floor and stamps it out with her foot. The fire wants fixing; she turns on so much fuel that it all runs down and over the floor; to terrify the patient she leaves the stove door open till the house is filled with smoke. The braid of her dress is loose; she catches that on the chairs and drags them after her. Her fingers are tied up with a rag and rolled with a black string; they have been scalded by hot water which she undertook to turn into the teapot. She brings another plate of food directly, and declares to the patient that she knows he will die if he don't eat something; so that the patient is annoyed and gets nervous, fever comes on and he gets no sleep the live-long night. Such a woman is the best in the world, and she does the very best she knows; but she makes a very poor nurse.

THE LAZY NURSE.

This kind "putters,' dreams and drawls; she never begins; she never ends. She has neither system nor smartness; no accurate idea of anything; if you undertake to tell her anything her mind wanders off, and she will begin to talk to you about a dozen different subjects. She starts off, to do something you tell her to do, as if she was in a great hurry, but her intellect seems to have left her, and lo! she has forgotten what you told her. She feebly moans her monotones, and brings you the wrong article. I feel sorry for this one.

THE CRUEL NURSE.

This kind will do her duty, but she does it by law and that without mercy. She will carry out the doctor's orders, but it lacks the right spirit. She fixes the medicine at the right time, and it must be taken forthwith. She changes the clothes no matter how it hurts. A little tenderness and compassion would improve this kind most wonderfully.

THE CARELESS NURSE.

This one forgets to give the medicine at the right time; also forgets the patient in many particulars. The soiled dishes are scattered around the room, and she lets the food stand for hours at the bedside after the patient has partaken of all he wants. The bed is full of crumbs and seldom made up; the fire burns low or goes out; the ashes are strewn all over the hearth. She means well and she does the very best she knows. Still she makes a very poor nurse.

THE FUSSY NURSE.

Now this one is liable to overdo everything. She intends to have everything just right. She runs in and out every few minutes—here she goes hither and yonder. She tires the patient nearly to death with her interrogations. "Now how do you feel? Won't you have a drink? Can't you eat something?" She raises his head, then tucks the bedclothes in here and there. She pins back the curtains; then she sweeps the floor. She brings the medicine, fixes the eatables; always on the go. She is too good to sit still, and yet her very goodness is damaging to the patient. She ought to be more quiet and take things more easy.

THE DISHONEST NURSE.

The very worst of all is the dishonest nurse. I have known some such nurses, who would eat all the food and drink all the wine, turn out the medicine, and then try to make me believe the patient took all I had left. But these poor creatures are very few, and we thank the Lord for it.

THE TATTLING NURSE.

A Tattler is an abomination, a weariness to the flesh. Of all the nurses this one is the first to be shunned. She is a curse and a great damage to all who are around her. She keeps the patient and everybody else in a perfect stew and worry. No person under her eye can feel secure. But thank the Lord, for humanity's sake, we seldom see this kind.

Every nurse should be a person who has good judgment and a full exercise of his or her senses; should have:

Sight—To read directions, and sometimes to read to amuse the patient.

Hearing—To catch the faintest whisper, and to avoid a great effort in speaking.

Feeling—To determine the change in temperature in the room, the heat of the body, the moisture or dryness of the skin, and to know when applications are to be made—when they are too cold or too hot—to see that all drafts are avoided when sponging or bathing the patient.

Smelling—To detect all effluvias or impurities that are in the room.

Taste—To determine the seasoning of the food.

A careful exercise of all the natural faculties, with a study of the principles of nursing, ought to make a competent person to care for the sick.

The Room for the Sick.

It is not every family who have a choice of rooms, but under all circumstances we must do the best we can. A room should be selected that is light and cheerful. The *head* of the bed should be placed to the *north*, if possible, as the currents of electricity in nature run from north to south. If the patient has some kind of fever or brain disorder, or some nervous disease, let the room be in some quiet part of the house, away from the family. If it is a bone broken or fracture from the result of some accident, then the patient should be near the rest of the family, for in such cases it is very often amusement for the patient to watch the movements of the rest. Avoid a room that is exposed to any kind of effluvia. Have the windows so that they can be let down at the top. The less furniture in the room the better, especially if the disease be infectious. Before putting the patient in the room see to it that it has been well aired, warmed and dried. First, light the fire and see that the chimney draws well. The best bed is a hair mattress, but clean straw or husks will answer very well. *Remember* that feather beds are not healthy; besides they are inconvenient, especially if the patient has a broken bone or fractured leg, and in wounds and burns—the patient is apt to sink down into holes. When the patient is to be changed and the party cannot get up, you can get the patient on the edge of the bed; now roll up against the patient all the bed clothes that you intend to change, have your clean sheets and blankets all ready; now spread them on the bed smooth and straight; now get your patient to roll over carefully on the clean sheets; now take off the dirty clothes, and then spread out the other half of the clean change. Now, don't you see, you have it all done nicely. If it is necessary to scour the room to purify it, wash it with hot water, after first adding a few cents' worth of chloride of lime, or some crude carbolic acid. Then dry the room thoroughly and it is ready.

Food and Drinks for the Sick.

It will be necessary for you to know how to prepare certain kinds of foods which the doctor may order for the patient. It is well that you should understand a few general principles that should govern the administration of food. First, then, solid food is seldom admissable, especially during acute diseases of any kind, for the reason that the stomach and digestive organs are not in a condition to furnish the fluids necessary for its comminution; hence, instead of digesting, it simply lies there and decomposes, which will give rise to irritation, and hence it will produce other serious complications. Second. The more severe the disease the more delicate and lighter the food should be diluted. Thus, in a high grade of fever or inflammation we should give whey, beef tea, extract of beef, milk punch, toast water, mutton broth, tapioca, chicken broth. Third. When there is great exhaustion, then the food should be all the more concentrated, and very nutritious. Then let us give the *Extract of Beef*, or beef essence as it is sometimes called, concentrated chicken or mutton broth, milk and cream. Fourth. In fevers or inflammatory diseases, give the food at the period of the day or night in which there is least vascular and nervous excitement, and never force it upon the patient if suffering from a high grade of fever. Fifth. Never give food in severe pain. Sixth. Then if the tongue is coated with a yellow coat, and bad taste in the mouth, with a feeling of weight and oppression in the stomach, it is better not to give food; or if given it should always be in a liquid form. Seventh. When the digestion is impaired and it becomes necessary to sustain life with food, it should be given in small quantities and at regular intervals, like medicine, every two or three hours. Eighth. In convulsions much care is required in keeping the patient from eating too much.

Recipes for Cooking.

BEEF TEA.

Take one pound of nice, tender steak, remove the fat, chop very fine, put it in a pint of cold water, stir it and let it soak one hour, then boil it ten minutes, strain it and season to suit the taste of the patient or your own judgment in case of great exhaustion and great debility of the digestive organs.

EXTRACT OF BEEF.

Take a Scotch ale *stone* bottle (it is best), scald it out so that you know it is clean; take one pound of nice, tender and fat beef steak; after removing the fat, chop it up fine, season it with a little salt and pepper, put it in the bottle, cork it up tight, then tie the cork down so that you know that it will not fly out with the heat and steam; now place the bottle into a *pot* of water and boil it for three hours. Remember you cannot cook it too much. When done and mostly used up the remaining liquor can be pressed out, then the bottle can be refilled with fresh meat and cooked for the next day. This preparation is very rich, with nutritious element; two tablespoonfuls at a dose for an adult is sufficient, repeated every two or three hours. A little can be poured out at a time and warmed on the stove as it is required. Keep the bottle well corked; if it is left open the extract will lose much of its strength, as well as its flavor.

CHICKEN JELLY.

Take half a raw chicken, pound it well with a mallet, bones and all, cover it over with cold water; heat it slowly in a covered vessel, let it simmer till the meat is thoroughly cooked, then strain the liquor through a coarse cloth; now season it to taste, return it to the stove and let it simmer ten minutes longer, skim it when cool and give it to the patient.

BARLEY WATER.

Take of pearl barley two ounces, boiling water two quarts, boil down to one quart and strain; a little lemon and sugar may now be added. This is a good drink in all inflammatory and eruptive diseases, scarlet fever, measles, small pox, etc.

RICE WATER.

Take of good rice two ounces, water two quarts, boil one and a half hours, then add sugar and nutmeg to suit the taste; use with milk. This an excellent diet for children.

ARROWROOT JELLY.

One cup of boiling water, two teaspoonfuls of Bermuda arrowroot; wet the arrowroot in a little cold water and rub smooth, then stir it into the hot water, which should be on the fire and boiling, with sugar already in it; stir until clear, then add one teaspoonful of lemon juice; now wet a cup with cold water and pour the jelly, and let it form. Eat with sugar and cream, if you like.

BARLEY JELLY.

Boil one quart of water, let it cool; take one-third of a loaf of bread (common size), slice it up and pare off the crust. Toast it to a light brown, put it in the water in a covered vessel and boil it gently till you find, on putting some in a spoon to cool, that it becomes a jelly; now strain it and cool; add sugar and lemon juice, or grate a little lemon peel as it is used.

OATMEAL GRUEL.

Two tablespoonfuls of oatmeal, one quart water, boil ten minutes and strain; salt and sugar to suit your taste.

CORNMEAL GRUEL.

Made the same way, using cornmeal instead of oatmeal.

OATMEAL WATER.

Take two ounces of oatmeal, one quart of water, stir up well, let stand till settled, then drink the water with ice in it, if you choose. This is an excellent drink for diarrhœa or in dysentery.

AGAIN—Take milk one pint, sheep's suet three ounces, corn starch half an ounce, cardamon seeds one ounce browned like you would coffee, then grind it very fine; after the other mixture is boiled gently for thirty minutes stir in the ground seed while it is yet hot; when cool it can be used as food and medicine. It is excellent. It will cure the very worst cases of dysentery or bloody flux. It does the work when the best of doctors fail.

BUTTERMILK PAP.

Take of fresh buttermilk four parts, water one part, mix and boil, then thicken with corn or oatmeal. Eat with butter and molasses.

WINE WHEY.

Heat a pint of new milk until it boils, at which moment pour in as much good wine as will curdle and clarify it; boil again, and set aside until the curd subsides; pour off the whey carefully and add two pints of boiling water and loaf sugar to suit the taste.

ORANGE WHEY.

Milk one pint, the juice of one orange with a portion of the rind; boil the milk, then add the orange juice; let stand till it coagulates, then strain. Both of the above are excellent for convalescent patients where there is weak digestion, for children or adults.

VEGETABLE SOUP.

Take one potato, one turnip, and one onion, with a little celery or celery seed; slice each, and boil one hour in a quart of water; season to taste; then pour the whole upon a piece of toast.

ELM-BARK JELLY.

Take two teaspoonfuls of finely pulverized elm bark and one pint of cold water; stir until a jelly is formed; sweeten with loaf sugar. This is excellent for all diseases of the throat and lungs, coughs, colds, etc. It is very nutritious.

FLAX-SEED LEMONADE OR COUGH SYRUP.

Four tablespoonfuls of whole flax seed, half an ounce horehound herb, one quart boiling water; let steep for three hours in a covered vessel and strain the juice from three roasted onions, the juice of two lemons; tincture of lobelia and ipecacuanha, of each three drachms; add sugar to sweeten; if too thick, add a little water. Partake of it freely; it is excellent for colds, coughs, throat or lung, as well as kidney trouble.

MILK PUNCH.

Take two fresh eggs, two tablespoonfuls loaf sugar; beat well together on a plate; add one pint of new milk, nutmeg and good brandy or whiskey to flavor it well. This is *par excellence* the best sustaining food in low grades of fever for children or adults. Alternate with the Extract of Beef, (see page 14,) patients will live on it for days and weeks.

The Little Infant.

"A babe in a house is the well-spring of happiness." The young husband steps about with a joyful air, with his head carried much higher than ever before; he feels proud. Why shouldn't he? He is proud of the title of Father, and the fond wife looks and smiles through her tears, feeling the pleasure of at last becoming a mother. Baby looks just like its father, except its hair and eyes—they resemble its mother; but it is a bonny little thing, a messenger of peace and a joy to all. But what shall we do with it? Well, we will tell you, but first we must tell you what is too often done in such cases: First, it is washed, then some spirits is rubbed on its head, then one or two caps, then some flannels are put on it, and it is dressed; now it must take a little something, for the dear little creature must be hungry—so a little whiskey, salt and molasses are mixed and brought and poured down its delicate little throat; next it must have physic—a little castor oil is given, then a little baby soup is mixed up and given, after which it is put to bed to sleep. But, alas, not to sleep, for now here is where the music begins, and all hands are engaged in the waltz. The baby cries, and cries, and frets, and nobody gets any peace in that house. But surely something must be done. "Why, I do wonder what ails it? It surely must be sick," says one; "The child has the colic," says another; then a dose of paregoric is given; then in a few moments a dose of soothing syrup is poured down, and if the crying ceases, it swoons away under the influence of the narcotic poison it has taken; now do go for the doctor, and when he arrives he finds it in a fit that has been produced by a reckless interference with nature. Now, all of this is cruel; yes, it is an abomination. It was not done intentionally, of course, but it don't help the baby, to say it was done in kindness.

Now, this is no imaginary picture. We have watched over hundreds of them, and, as they are not able to speak for themselves, you must allow us to speak for them and vindicate their claims. So we will proceed to give you a few hints: First, there is no oil, whiskey or salt needed, but if you will just keep them away you will soon learn that there is no necessity of giving paregoric or soothing syrup either to cure the colic. If the baby has a mother living, the first supply of milk from her will be better than anything else, and it is just what

God designed it should have. It is no matter if the baby does not get anything to eat for the first thirty-six hours. No baby yet has ever died for want of food the first two days of its life; but there have been hundreds, ah, yes, thousands, killed by the reckless interference, by giving such miserable stuff as we have mentioned. If you do not abuse your little infant, its stomach will require no treatment.

Having now rid your minds of this nonsense, you will next want to know what should be done. This is what we will endeavor to tell you: First, prepare all of its clothing with little tapes, having a a needle and thread handy to tack it with, instead of pins; wash your baby with a little soft water and mild castile soap; use a little glycerine, rubbing it over the body to dissolve the oily particles, then wash it off and dry the skin; use no spirits of any kind; do not fasten the clothes too tight; use no cap on the head, and give it *nothing*. By placing it to the mother, if it can be borne, it will be sufficient, but if you cannot resist the temptation long enough for nature to supply the proper nourishment, give it a little milk and warm water, sweetened with sugar of milk; then, with its body clean and warm, and its breath sweetened with angel purity and sweetness, lay it away in a warm, cosy nest, then you can sit down in comfort and see it rest easy, in a manner that will soon convince you that you have done right. But, if the mother should not furnish the proper supply in three or four days, then you can furnish it with the artificial nourishment, properly prepared. Children, as they grow older, may require food. The milk of some mothers becomes impoverished, and, consequently, the child grows poor and is never satisfied; then, in that case, take a little bread, arrowroot and sugar, and simmer in a little water until it is quite smooth, then add milk until it is the proper thickness; sweeten a little, and give it to your baby. Remember, however, that the natural food is the mother's milk, and any deviation from that standard of natural constituents is, consequently, more or less injurious, as the babies are not always hungry when they cry; it may be a pin, a tight compression on some part of the body, or it may be sickness. Babies are like older people—creatures of *habit*—and it is astonishing how soon they will form a habit. If you teach it the habit of being rocked to sleep, then that is what it wants when it cries and desires to sleep; therefore, you can teach it good habits as well as bad ones. You can teach it the habit of cleanliness, with very little trouble and regular attendance every day. Just try it, and be convinced; if you will, your baby will be healthy and sweet. How often have we seen a mother rocking her baby to sleep, and then when she tries to lay it down it is as wide awake as ever? We have seen them try this a half dozen times or more before succeeding. Lay it down awake, and when nature requires sleep it will soon come. But this habit must be taught from the beginning, if not you will have considerable trouble to antagonize the habit by and by.

TEETHING.

More children die passing this period of their lives than at any other time; just when they have began to grow so interesting. Up to this period in their lives they have always been so healthy; they have not been sick a day; they are so fat and healthy, and look so sweet; they have began to pull on the love strings, which wind so tight about the mother's heart. But, ah, me; they are beginning to cut their teeth, and are so sick. Now, if we can be the means of teaching mothers how to save their children from the grave, while they are passing through this critical period of their lives, we will feel that this little book has accomplished its purpose, and our life has not been lived in vain.

When a child is teething, there is a heavy pressure upon the gums from the teeth forcing their way through; this, of course, produces irritation and inflammation of the gums; they become very tender and sore to the touch. This acts upon the nervous system and is sometimes followed by high fever; the stomach and bowels are all out of order, and the child is fretful and sick. If the bowels become relaxed, and it vomits up its food, etc., do not fly to your soothing syrup, or your paregoric and laudanum. One drop of laudanum, or five drops of paregoric, or half a teaspoonful of soothing syrup have each been known to kill an infant. Do not, we beg of you, suffer anybody to ever give your child those medicines, but use your little simple remedies which you know all about—at least you know they will do no harm.

If you fail to furnish sufficient milk for the child, or if it has began to eat food, be careful what you give it to eat. Do not give it any green vegetables or green fruit, but resort to your Extract of Beef, Oatmeal Water, Milk Punch, &c.; (see pages 14, 16 and 17,) they will be sufficient to carry your child through safely. Keep the child warmly clad; change its garments every time the weather changes; if it is broken out with the heat, bathe its body occasionally with a little soda water, (such soda as you use for baking purposes,) wipe it dry and dust its body with a little cream of tartar. Occasionally give your baby a little lime water in its milk; also, give it a piece of nice dried beef in its hand to suck—cut it in a long, round strip so that it cannot swallow it, and thus be choked to death. If you will follow these rules, you will seldom ever have to call a physician; but if they all fail, you may call a physician who has age and experience in the treatment of little children, whom you have confidence in.

When the teeth are coming through avoid giving it hard substances to bite upon, for it breaks the enamel upon the teeth and they are apt to decay. The best thing is an India rubber ring, which you can get at the drug store. Wash it off clean, then spread some molasses upon it, and the child will work upon this with perfect pleasure and safety. But if the teeth are tedious in coming through, and the gums become much swollen and inflamed, you had better take it to the doctor and insist upon him to cut the gums, or, better still, to a good dentist, who will scarify the gums over each tooth. We have done this many times, and have been astonished to see how quickly the stomach and bowel trouble would all pass away, and the child be apparently well in a very few days. When the child gets old enough to walk, do not make it stand too long at a time upon its feet. If one child walks at a certain age, it is no reason why another should. If you force your child to walk you run the risk of bending its limbs.

Some people are in the habit of scaring their children about "the doctor! the doctor will come and cut your ears off. He will pull your teeth out." Now, this is all wrong, to scare your child about anything, no matter what, especially about the doctor. If you do not want your child to be timid and a coward all through its life, never allow anybody to try to scare your child. How can the physician, under such circumstances, find out the condition of the tongue or the state of the pulse when the little child is almost frightened to death and trembling with fear? Do not terrify the child in this way. Impress the idea that when he comes he will cure them if they are sick, and is a friend to them when well; then the child will learn to be calm as well as trustful; besides, they will be much easier restored to health. When they have confidence the medicine has a much better effect. There is a great difference between a grown person and a child when sick, for an adult has a dread of death, and, in many instances, a greater dread of the consequences after death. Hence, he submits very readily to treatment in the hope of living longer; while the child has no fear of death nor the consequences after death, for its mind is too young yet to be doctrinated into the false ideas of the condition of life beyond the grave. But the child only dreads, and knows nothing of anything only its present pain. Children, therefore, if not too weak to bear it, should be amused with toys, and pictures; give them a slate and pencil, a doll or a pet dog, a kitten, anything to cheer up their little spirits and give the best chances for a recovery.

Eating.

The brain is interested in the process of digestion. If it is excited or over-taxed, or even over-vexed, it will not stimulate the stomach to work till it is rested. Never eat when you are mad, fatigued, or exhausted. Drink a little gruel if you are very hungry, then wait till you are rested before you take a full meal. Always give the stomach time to rest between meals. Always eat regular, and not by piece-meals. Frequent eating, as well as too frequent nursing of children, soon weakens the stomach and liver, and brings on dyspepsia and other kinds of diseases.

EAT SLOWLY.—Rapid eating, and drinking so much while eating, is the curse of this nation. It produces palpitation of the heart, vertigo, headache, neuralgia, nervous debility, spinal irritation, rheumatism, premature old age. Chew your food thoroughly, drink but little while eating, take plenty of time; don't be in a hurry. Take thirty minutes' time to eat your meals. Remember that stomach bitters will not chew your food for you. You are better off without such stuff.

COMMON LAMENTATION.—What is the cry of our fast-going people? "My food does not digest;" this is the saying all over America. "My poor head aches half the time;" so exclaim our young ladies. "My lungs are the best part of me," which you can hear most any day, "but my liver is diseased and torpid." This is a popular complaint. "And my bowels are slow and sluggish." Such miserable lamentations ascend from all the most fertile portions of this glorious continent. But we feel glad that there is an awakening in the direction of physiological knowledge and universal improvement, and the final triumph will surely be: The triumphant conquest of individual man over all enemies to his bodily ease and mental tranquility.

Is it not worthy of particular notice that the majority of people who, as invalids, incessantly complain in the department of digestion, are the most constant violators of physiological law? If, however, any person should flatter him or herself that he or she can go on violating the conditions of *Health*, and, at the same time, by simply yielding to the self-restoring mercies of his spiritual constitution, recover all his original vigor and bloom, his disappointment will be complete. Mother Nature is just as loving and as just as Father God; but they do not, because they cannot, guarantee impunity from the effects of violation. All the medical isms and myths and pathies from Hippocrates down to the last nostram cannot perform the pardoning act. There is no infallible remedy, so you might as well pass the word all around the world—there is no specific for any human transgression. Let every eye read it, let every ear hear it, and inscribe it in fadeless characters upon the Temple of Health.

Lung Life.

Deprive the lungs of heaven's invisible air—shut off the supply of the vivifying principle of the Divine Infinitude—and the whole beautiful machinery will stop. *Remember this*, that the best food in the the universe could give you no strength unless first baptized in the spirit of the atmosphere. Air is the Universal! Thank the Lord that it cannot be fenced in by legislative enactment. But it can and often is kept by *ignorance* or inattention out of the lungs of invalids. Some persons seem to be afraid to expand their lungs to their utmost capacity for fear something will break and let out the stream of life. Of course, dear reader, you know that any sudden and violent conduct will be attended with a great percentage of risk. Begin deliberately to practice daily, therefore, and you will find that the air is impregnated with an electric energy which pervades, refreshes, quickens and energizes every part of your physical temple. *Remember*, your food cannot digest, neither can your blood circulate, without the electric fire of the air; neither can a particle of food strengthen you without it. Without the living energy of the air, which is obtained only through the lungs, no diet could be made universally nutritious. Salivary juice, as it pours out from the little springs on either side of the cheeks and mouth, could do nothing without the vivifying electricity of the air. The gastric fluids—although loaded with its inherent pepsin and the acids, lactic, hydrochloric, etc., etc.—could accomplish nothing without a constant supply of nerve-energy. The lungs must absorb the electricity of the measureless immensity; otherwise nothing strong can occur, but death and transformation will hasten into the temple.

Singular Physiological Facts.

The shortest route to health is through the lungs. Small lungs—small minds; or large lungs and bad air; large minds and few thoughts. The old-fashioned orthodox churches were built and kept as tight as drums during service. The effect was manifest in narrow creeds and doleful doctrines concerning God and man. In this connection we are reminded of Florence Nightingale, the noble nurse who voluntarily went to the Crimean war to bind up the bleeding soldiers. She says: "An extraordinary fallacy is the dread of night air. What air can we breathe at night but night air. The choice is from between pure night air from without and foul night air from within. Most people prefer the latter. An unaccountable choice. What will they say if it is proved to be true that fully one-half of the diseases we suffer from are occasioned by people sleeping with their windows shut. An open window most nights in the year can never hurt anyone. This is not to say that the light is not necessary for recovery. In great cities night air is the best and purest, out of the twenty-four hours. We could better understand shutting the windows in towns during the day than during the night, for the sake of the sick; for the absence of smoke and dust, as well as the quietude, all tend to make the night air the best for airing the sick. It is impossible to keep well, and have good digestion, without the pure air, and plenty of it; it is impossible to think large, manly, beautiful and virtuous thoughts, while respiring in an atmosphere of stagnation and consequent corruption. People who sleep in close, ill-ventilated rooms are forever dreaming a set of monotonous dreams, loaded with vicious pictures, and animated by strangers or demons, made from the confined air. Idiots breathe superficially; they seldom respire like an intelligent mind. Timid persons inhale small quantities of air. The coward has a narrow chest, and he only uses the upper portion of his lungs. Why does the strongest horse always have the broadest and deepest chest? The mind cannot expand and improve, morally and intellectually, unless the lungs be large and full, and constantly and plentifully supplied with air fresh from the vestige of immensity; no health can be maintained in a confined atmosphere; no exalted thoughts; no spiritual preceptions.

PROCESS OF DIGESTION.

The Gastric Methods. The reasons in favor of full and intelligent respiration are numerous and easily understood. Chyle is the last result of fundamental digestion. But in itself, chyle has no power to promote growth, give strength, or repair the waste of the body. It is the successor to chyme. Chyme is manufactured from the food in the first part of digestion. It is first manufactured by the stomach into a pulpy mass, impregnated or charged with electricity of the vital kind. But when it passes downward into the lower stomach, or duodenum, the pancreatic fluids and the bile at once combine with it, thereby adding a positive element by which the chyme is transformed into a milk-white liquid (the chyle) which, with the residum, flows steadily into and through all the small intestines. What next? The numerous mesenteric glands, with the lacteal vessels, commence their work of forming incipient eggs from out the chylic fluids; the unchylified portions (the residum) meantime passes onward into the large and lower bowels, and is then rejected, together with the broken-down blood globules, in the shape of bile and relative excretions. This material is wholly excrementious.

Now the thoracic duct, so-called, attracts the chyle from the lacteal passages and mesenteric glands, and pours it into a vein which, from behind the collar-bone, discharges its contents into the positive side of the heart; there the blood is mixed with the negative portions of the venous blood, which is no more nutritious than the chyle; neither can it give strength nor repair waste.

THE PURIFYING ORDEAL OF THE BLOOD.

How is this accomplished? By means of the pure air of space. Yes; when Heaven's devout breath enters the air-chambers the chyle is at once converted into nutritious blood, baptized to the multifarious necessities of the arterial system, while at the same time the cold venous blood is unloaded of its dead-burdens in the form of carbonic gas and useless water. Carbon is the principal element of decay and death, yet it is very essential to life and a good conductor to electricity. So, therefore, the heart very wisely and energetically throws both the chyle and venous blood upon the entire responsibility of the lungs; so that when the invisible air is drawn by deep breathing into the pulmonary structure the divine life also enters, whereby the chyle is changed as by magic into the constructive principle for the soul's good, whereby the newly purified blood is re-baptized and confirmed into the ways of righteousness; it hastens upon its mission of benevolence to all parts of the physical temple. Now, my dear reader, we feel that we have put this question in a light that you may understand fully the process of digestion, as well as the importance of lung life in health, as well as the necessity of ventilation in the sick room; so that you may better and more fully understand us when we speak upon the different conditions, on the pages of this little book, of How to Live, and what to do in all circumstances in disease and misfortune which may come upon you. For you must remember that nearly all diseases can be traced to the stomach and lungs, as the first origin from improper air and bad digestion.

REMEDY FOR CONSTIPATION.

Many persons who are troubled with biliousness, jaundice, sick-headache, fever, chills, etc., which is a constant persistent inactivity of the bowels. Dear reader, pills and cathartic medicines will not cure you, for thousands have tried it, over and over again. The old complaint is still lingering with you, and has been for years. We will tell you how you can, with a very simple medicine and a judicious use of diet, cure yourself of it, and of all the above ills, and keep you free from those troubles, When the system is clogged and surcharged with broken-down blood of wasted tissue, semi-oxygenated fluids (out of which all manner of corruption, jaundice, bilious sick-headache, melancholy, fever and chills, are brought forth.

REMEDY.—Take plenty of time to eat your meals, chew your food well; no meat, no coffee, no hot cakes oftener than twice per week. Plenty of all kinds of fruit sauce for breakfast and supper, cracked wheat, graham bread or mush, or oatmeal, baked potatoes, vegetables of all kinds. If you will live in this way you will be astonished how soon you will get rid of all those bilious troubles; not one, but all will pass away from you, never to return.

For immediate relief—Take a tablespoonful of Indian meal or graham flour in a tumbler of water before breakfast, quite early in the morning; perhaps several doses will be necessary, together with our sovereign remedy.

Take two drachms each of tincture of mandrake (podophylin), tincture of Turkey rhubarb and tincture of nux vomica, one ounce of fluid extract of Cascara Sagrada of Park, Davis & Co.'s manufacture, tablespoonful of powdered willow charcoal, orange peel and cloves, well powdered, of each one tablespoonful; put all in one pint of good Holland gin, add half a pint of water, half pound of sugar. Shake it well. Dose: Teaspoonful half hour after each meal and one on going to bed. Take it for a week or more, or longer if required. Keep this medicine in your house, and you will never need any other for all those bilious troubles which trouble more or less one out of every family.

NEURALGIA.

This is another malady which afflicts the human family. But if the system is much clogged up, as described in bilious conditions (see page 26) it may be necessary to take a good bath, first soaking the feet in a bucket of hot water, after first adding a tablespoonful of ground mustard, drinking some hot ginger tea, or, better still, a tea made from the smart weed. This is excellent. Now go to bed, add a few bottles of hot water to the feet and around the limbs. Pile on now the blankets and the comforts several thicknesses, and after commencing to sweat keep it up for thirty or forty minutes. Don't be afraid of sweating too long, for its not going to hurt you. Now, while you are sweating go to rubbing and scratching yourself, You will be astonished at the amount of the gluey matter that you can roll off from your body. Of this you must get off all that you can while you are sweating under the cover, as it is the only time and place that it will come off. Have some friend to sponge your body off with a warm, wet towel and soap while you are yet under the covers. When you get through the sweat, you can be sponged off with a little warm water, wiped dry and rubbed hard with the towel, Or, better still, give the body a brisk rubbing with the bare hands for twenty minutes. With this treatment, together with the following remedy, we have never failed to cure neuralgia permanently. It is as follows: *Neuralgia*—Sal amonia in one ounce of camphor-water to be taken teaspoonful at a time, and the dose repeated several times at intervals of five minutes till the pain is relieved, then prolong the intervals. If, however, the pain is very acute and severe, for external use you can use the following, no matter where the pain is located—neck, face, teeth or ears: Wine of opium, 30 drops, sulphuric ether half a drachm; fluid extract of belladonna, fluid extract gelseminum, of each one drachm, one ounce of lavender water. Mix all together, saturate a cotton cloth with the mixture and apply it for an hour or more over the region of the pain.

Bath.

Some convenient apparatus should be kept in every dwelling for bathing purposes. Baths are used both in health and disease. Bathing or sponging is indispensable, for cleanliness is godliness. Wash the skin all over at least twice a week. Use a little castile soap and then wipe dry, having the room the right temperature. Every family could have a cosy little bath room by itself, with very little expense, to be used in health or sickness. By having a wooden box made with a door to it large enough for a person to sit on a stool—something like a piano stool, that could be raised or lowered at will—for the bather to sit on; the bath box so arranged that the head could be outside when the door is closed close around the neck. With such a bath box as this, no one would need any other kind of bath fixtures about the house; for with this kind of a bath box there could be nearly every different kind of bath given that would be required for any purpose whatever; such as the alcoholic vapor bath, steam bath, electrical bath, medicated vapor bath, shower bath, spray bath, etc., etc., by having a reservoir, some distance from the bath box, holding sufficient warm or tepid water for the purpose, with a rubber hose running from the reservoir to the bath box. In this way you could take your alcoholic sweat by placing a lamp with a large wick made for that purpose, and set it under your stool and take a good sweat; first, with your feet placed in a bucket of hot water, after all of which, you could shampoo yourself with soap, then spray yourself off from the rubber hose, which should be supplied with a nice spray-fixture on the end of the hose, filled full of very fine holes for the water to pass through, and hung up on the inside of the bath box—some place handy. Then, after shampooing your body with soap you could have an attendant to turn on the water so you could spray yourself off while sitting in the box all shut up. Now this is one of the most delightful baths that ever was given, and does far more good for the sick or well than a bath taken in any other way, as you can have the water any temperature you desire, and change it at will. In this case you see the *fresh* water runs on you all the while and passes off into your *waste* pipe, which, of course, should be attached to the bottom of the bath box. If people would only so arrange their bath houses or boxes in this way, so that the bathers could have the water run on them by means of a fine spray and pass off, it would be more scientific. It is very much better than lying in the water, for the reason that, in this way, you receive all the electrical and magnetic elements that are in the water, and thus your bath acts like a tonic to the human body, giving strength and vigor ; while lying in the water the old way is not so cleansing; besides, if you lie in the water over twenty-five minutes, it is weakening in its effects.

Alcoholic sweat baths given in this way, from the dry, hot air from the alcoholic lamp, (for you should use no other kind of heat for this purpose but alcohol), is a better method for curing rheumatism and neuralgia than all other medicines in the world, for it will cure them every time without fail, but it must be repeated two or three times per week. Try it.

The best way to give a baby a bath when it is sick and afraid of the water, is to take a small blanket and wring it out from warm water, spread it over the mother's lap, and lay the baby on the wet blanket and wrap it all up, and wrap a dry blanket over that to keep out the cold air. Keep the child in this condition for thirty or forty minutes, then unwrap it and change it to a warm, dry sheet, and wrap it up again till it has all dried off. You can, while wrapped up in the sheet, rub it dry with the sheet, then you can change its clean clothes. This method can be repeated as often as desired with safety, and it is very efficient in many of the ills that are incident to children. However, you are to remember that in all cases of this kind that the room must be warm ; no draft from the doors and windows while administering the bath.

THE FOOT BATH.

This bath is very efficient for many purposes. For headaches or for a sudden cold, this is often used on going to bed. A large bucket, or any kind of a deep vessel, is used. Fill it up with as hot water as can well be borne, place the feet in it and throw a quilt over the limbs and lap to keep the heat in, and sit with the feet in this water for 30 minutes, or longer if desired. As the water cools there can be hot water added occasionally so as to keep the water as hot as can be borne. If the patient is troubled with cold feet, there can be a tablespoonful of ground mustard added and well mixed with the water beforehand. If you should wish to sweat after the bath, you should drink some hot teas while taking the bath, such as ginger tea, or the smart weed, or a hot lemonade with a little whisky or capsicum (red pepper) added to it. To get the full benefit of such a bath you should go immediately to bed and have some hot irons to the feet, and cover up well. Keep still till you get into a sweat.

THE HIP, or SITZ BATH.

Sufficient water should be placed in a tub to cover the hips and lower portion of the abdomen. When the patient is in a sitting posture the water can be made to any temperature to suit the immediate indications. And the patient should remain in the bath the length of time indicated by the physician. Most all physicians prescribe this bath for quite a number of diseases. We would add that in case of painful or even suppression of the monthlies, this bath is very good. Sometimes we order this and the foot bath also, (as described on page 29), with the feet in the bucket of water, while at the same time you sit in the tub of water.

Fevers.

In the management of fevers, no matter of what kind or by what name it is called by the attendant physician, the nurse should know how to manage the patient to subdue the fever before it gets to such a high grade as to become threatening and dangerous to life. Here is where the sponge bath is always practicable, at whatever time of the day or night. When the fever is the highest then is the time that the patient should be sponged off with tepid water, not too cold, not hot. Part of the body can be gone over at a time, generally first the head and face, then one arm laid bare, then the other, then the breast, neck and bowels, then one leg, then the other; cover up the body as you go; then have the patient turn over on the side while you can sponge the back and limbs clear to the feet. This mode can be repeated every hour while the fever lasts, taking care that you do not sponge the patient after the fever has gone down.

Remember, that there is never any danger of any body taking cold in giving a sponge bath while the fever is on; NEVER.

Again, remember, that, in all cases of fever, no matter what, the head should be kept cool by occasionally bathing the head and face with the bare hand wet in water. This can be repeated often while the fever runs high; while, at the same time the feet and lower extremities should be watched very closely and kept warm day and night, even if it must be done with hot irons or jugs of hot water, or wrapped up with hot flannels, heated by the stove. *Follow* these rules closely and nearly every case of fever can be controlled, and the patient made well in a very short time.

RULES TO OBSERVE.

Rule 1—Fever patients should have the right kind of nutritious food to keep up and sustain the *vital forces*. The food should consist of beef extract, chicken or mutton broth, milk punch, etc., made as dricted on pages 14, 15, 17. This food must be given at intervals of from two to three hours apart, only a little at a time. Great quantities of food must not be forced upon the patient. Patients never require very much food when sick. Never disturb or wake your patient up to give them medicine or food, unless they are under the influence of narcotic medicines, when it is known that they will fall asleep immediately afterwards, as sleep will do your patient more good than medicine; but watch them. As soon as they wake up be ready to give the medicines with the least disturbance about it, that they may get quiet and go to sleep again, regardless if it is over the time that it should have been given if they had been awake.

Rule 2—See to it that the room is well ventilated. If it is winter time the room should be kept 60 to 70 deg. Fahrenheit, unless during the time the fever is the highest. In summer time there is not much danger of the cold air, if you have plenty of clothes to regulate the temperature of the body. But the lungs must have fresh air and plenty of it.

Rule 4—Do not go from the cold air to the bedside of the sick; especially if the patient is in a perspiration, or the patient has rheumatism; for the skin is very sensitive, and you had better wait in a warm room first till you get warm. No person has any idea of the pain and suffering of this disease unless they have had it themselves. Every joint is racked with pain, and the least touch of cold air or fingers adds to the suffering. Even the banging of a door, the shutting of a window, or the squeaking of a shoe or a boot, is but adding agony to the patient, and must be avoided.

Rule 4—Do not have old bottles setting around. When you are through with the bottle that has been prescribed throw away the medicine and wash out your bottle, and set it away. It is best not to keep medicines over for another case of sickness, because it is never wanted.

Rule 5. To change the dress of a patient—Much distress is often caused by not properly understanding just how to proceed to get the arms in and out of the sleeves, and is often attended with difficulty. If the infliction is likely to continue. First, rip the sleeves open, then tack on some strings so that the sleeve can be tied. This will not injure the garment and it can be sewed up again when needed.

Rule 6—There is a secret in handling a broken bone or a sore limb. Never take hold with the points of your thumb and finger as though you were afraid of it; but take a firm grasp, or slip your hand under and let the limb lie in the palm of your hand, then support it with your thumb and finger. All nervous handling produces fear in the patient; while the patient always feels safe in the firm grasp and a steady nerve.

The Home Medicine Chest.

Every family has more or less medicine about their house; but usually, however, they are kept carelessly sitting around in no place in particular. It is well to have some small box, with a lock on it, and always kept in some convenient place. It would be useless for every house to keep a drug store; but it is always well enough to keep a few reliable medicines, such as you would be likely to use in a case of emergency. But let me entreat you, never do you keep or buy any patent medicines, the ingredients of which are not known to you. There has been more damage produced by them than good accomplished; and, for the most part, they have been put up by ignorant pretenders, whose sole object is to get your money. Keep your castor oil, sweet oil, a vial of laudanum, a little tincture of lobelia, syrup of ipecac, spirits of camphor, a bottle of glycerine and a vial of syrup of rhubarb. Keep in your chest a roll of lint, a roll of linen, a piece of flannel, some sticking plaster. Have your physician put you up a bottle of medicine for burns and scalds, and have a place for it in your chest. These are some of the medicines that every family should keep on hand; not too many—only those which you know how to use. And for obvious reasons they should always be kept by themselves where they could be had at a moment's notice—all well labeled that you may make no mistake.

Hemorrhage.

BLEEDING, AND HOW TO STOP IT.

Many a fond mother has had a terrible fright by her child running in with its face and clothes all smeared over with blood. It is astonishing to see what a big mark a very little blood will make. But then it is no wonder that bleeding will produce fright; animals will instinctively rush to the spot where one of their kind is bleeding to death. Blood is the life, and where there is much loss of it life is endangered. Now, there is something about the structure of the body that everybody should understand; indeed, a full knowledge of the entire structure of the human body should be acquired by everyone. It is to be hoped that this knowledge will be one of the fundamental branches taught in our public schools at no distant day. At least every child should be taught this important knowledge. They should be as familiar with the bones and their structure and uses, all the blood vessels, their origin and course, as they are of the rivers and lakes of the country; for no one can afford to be ignorant of the situation of the blood vessels; because some day, in the course of their lives, it may be a question with them of life and death, or that of some one of their friends. Accidents may happen to anyone. If the body is torn, cut or injured in any way, some one of the important blood vessels may be involved, and death may be the rusult in a very few moments, simply because no one present may have obtained the knowledge which they might have possessed with a very little study. Therefore it is very hard for us to give you rules to stop bleeding, for we do not expect everyone who reads this little book to understand anatomy. We cannot tell you as we would were you acquainted with the circulatory system; yet, if you will follow us through, what we do say we can give you a fair understanding of it.

BLEEDING FROM THE NOSE.

Occasionally we find a person bleeding from the nose; that is quite troublesome. The cause is generally concealed in the nervous system—*debility* of the nervous system. Loss of nervous force is the usual cause of hemorrhage, whether 'from the lungs, anus, nose, stomach or other parts of the body. Therefore, the true remedy consists in whatever restores vigor to the nervous system. Hamamelis (witch hazel) bark or pulverized borax applied within the nostrils will stop the bleeding very soon. In the meantime cold water should be poured upon the wrists and back of the neck until the parts are very much reduced in temperature, thus arresting the rush of blood to the head. Also, if you feel that the bleeding is going to commence, press on the large veins on either side of the throat, rubbing downwards gently.

BLEEDING ABOVE THE EAR.

If there is a wound above the ear, on either side of the head, place your finger about a quarter of an inch in front of the ear, upon the side injured, and press hard on your finger, as this point will be on the blood vessel that carries the blood from the heart up along the temple to the side of the head.

BLEEDING BELOW THE EYES.

All of the small *arteries* that carry the blood to the outside of the face, nose, lips and muscles of the face, spring from one main artery that passes over the under jaw about half-way from the angle to the point of the chin. Therefore, if you will place a nickle on your thumb over the lower edge of the jawbone you will at once arrest the bleeding.

BLEEDING FROM A WOUND IN AN ARM.

Grasp the arm about two inches below the arm-pit; press tightly upon that portion which lies next to the body and a little in front of the center of the arm-pit. Or you can make a roll or pad and place on the artery at this point, and tie a handkerchief around the part tightly, just below the arm-pit. Treated in this way will check all bleeding *below* this point till you can send for your physician to come and tie the artery and dress the wound properly and as it should be.

BLEEDING FROM WOUNDS IN THE LEG OR FOOT.

Lie down and support the limb above the head of the body. Now press upon the large artery which lies in front of the thigh, about mid-way of the leg, just below the groin. Fix a roll or pad, (just as directed to fix the pad to stop the bleeding of the arm), or if you are in the field by yourself, and should get a severe cut with the scythe or some other sharp instrument, no matter what, just take a handful of dry earth and clasp it to the wound and hold it tightly there with the hand till you can get assistance.

BLEEDING FROM THE STOMACH.

It is frightful to see any one vomiting blood, and it is quite dangerous; but not always as dangerous as it appears. Sometimes it is a question whether it is from the stomach or from the lungs. The blood from the stomach is darker in its color than the blood from the lungs, and it is frequently mixed with food and stringy and ropy.

REMEDY.—Give two teaspoonfuls of vinegar, or lemon juice in a little cold water, and repeat it every half hour till the bleeding stops, or till your physician comes. You can also give a little cracked ice, if you have it, and nothing more, unless you understand medicine.

BLEEDING FROM THE LUNGS.

You will know that the blood is from the lungs from it being constantly coughed up instead of vomiting; besides it is a scarlet color instead of being a dark color like that from the stomach, and it is frothy in its nature. Keep the shoulders raised pretty high by pillows; sponge the chest off with cold water and a little vinegar; make no exertion by talking; keep quiet; give the patient just a little bit of salt, half a teaspoonful at a dose, taken dry, and repeat it often in small doses. These are the only means at hand to be used by the common people, and many times they are the best that can be used when they do the work. The other agents belong to the doctor, and it requires an education and experience to use them successfully and with safety.

Wounds.

Wounds become dangerous more from their position than from their size. A small punctured wound may be more dangerous than a large cut; or, a small wound in a certain place may be more dangerous, while a large cut or wound in some other spot may not be attended with any danger whatever. If it be dark colored blood and flows with regularity, you may be able to manage it: but if it spurts out with little *jets*, however small the wound may be, you must use the same means to stop it as directed in chapter on how to stop bleeding, (by compress and bandage), and then send for your doctor at once. Cuts on the head, in the hair, cannot be dressed with a plaster. They may be dangerous even when you do not think so.

WOUNDS from splinters, nails, or from glass, must not be closed immediately. You must let the doctor see them.

BROKEN BONES AND DISLOCATIONS.

Of course you could not expect us to give you a treatise how to remedy this difficulty, for this could not be done in so small a book. We can only say that broken bones are easily detected by the patient not being able to raise the limb, by its bending or grating sound between where there are no joints. You may not be able to detect it, whether it is a dislocation, a fracture or a broken bone. Unless you are quite sure it is a case of out-of-joint you had better not undertake to jerk or pull it. Wait till the surgeon comes. Always take the safe side.

Infectious Diseases.

These are propagated by a specific of contagion, which gains access to the blood, thereby generating a virous in the system. They are contracted by inhalation of gaseous exhalations from patients suffering from diseases, or from the discharged materials from the lungs, skin or bowels. The atmosphere in neighborhoods may be so impregnated with this specific poison as to cause what is known as an EPIDEMIC.

When a quantity of contageous matter, however small, is introduced into the blood of a healthy person, it will be propagated into the blood, and the disease is the result. You must never undertake the treatment of these diseases yourself; better employ a good physician and a good nurse, and this will be enough for you to know that you have supplied the best means at your command. When the skin begins to peel off, if it is a child, you will find it constantly picking at the nose, lips, teeth, or finger nails. It is a curious fact, how they will interest themselves for hours, picking at themselves till they bleed, without seeming to feel the least pain ; nor is it any use for you to find fault with them, or even threaten them, for it will do no good; it seems to be a part of the disease. Your only remedy is to place mittens upon the hands. After scarlet fever or small-pox, the room, together with all of its furniture, should be thoroughly disinfected. To accomplish this, cleanse the floor with hot water and lime, or carbolic acid ; close the room air-tight, after removing everything wet or moist from it, and then you can burn flour of sulphur ; this can be done by placing an iron kettle, with legs to it, in the center of the room. Or better still: Heat the kettle sufficiently hot to burn sulphur in it, then throw or sprinkle two or three ounces of sulphur in the kettle, then hasten out and close the door tight; let this remain closed for three or four hours, then it can be opened and aired for several days; then if you should whitewash the walls, your room would be as pure as it ever was.

WHOOPING-COUGH.

This disease does not show itself in two or three days. At first the symptoms are merely that of a slight cold; the child has a short, dry cough, particularly upon food being taken; this will continue, perhaps, for a week, or longer, before you will notice any other particular symptoms arise. Now, the fit of coughing is preceded by a convulsive drawing in of the breath, which, as it rushes into the lungs, causes the peculiar WHOOP; the cough lasts for a minute or two, then generally ends with vomiting; the breathing is then quiet for a time, and the child is comparatively at ease, until the next spasm of coughing comes on. Children under two years of age are generally exposed to more danger in this disease than older ones. However, if the child has convulsive coughs, we would advise you to seek for medical advice. Our late medical progress has done much towards a successful management of this disease, the Eclectic in particular, to which class of practitioners the author feels proud to belong. They have done much, of late years, by the use of newly discovered remedies, to mitigate the suffering from whooping-cough, and many children are cured without going through the usual prolonged and allotted time for the disease. But we feel that we cannot give you a special treatment here for this complicated disease. It is not the purpose of this little book to advise you to handle medical agents which you know nothing about; but to point out to you the true road for you to follow to gain your health. Besides we feel opposed to anybody handling medical agents without a thorough knowledge of medicine. In mild cases, and with best care, the following medicine, red pepper tea sweetened with honey, with a few drops of tincture of lobelia, used as a gargle several times a day, will be all that is necessary in most of these cases; but you must protect the chest with suitable thick clothing and keep the feet warm and dry. You must not resort to the usual cough medicines and syrups, for they will do no good and many times produce injury.

CROUP.

Croup is a very alarming disease, and well it may be; for it requires immediate treatment in many cases to save life. Sometimes it runs a very rapid course and destroys life in a very few hours. We will tell you how you can recognize it. It commences with a short dry cough; but the cough always sounds hoarse, then the breathing is increased and labored—there is a pecular rasping, or grating, or choking sound, which seems to proceed from the throat. Now, if you have got a case of this kind on your hands you must immediately go to work. Here we can give you a reliable treatment that will always do good service:

Tincture of ipecac	1 drachm.
Tincture of lobelia seed	1 "
Tincture of aconite root	10 drops.
Powdered niter	4 drachms.
Bromide of potassium	20 grains.
Glycerine	4 ounces.
Distilled water	1 ounce.

Mix all together and shake well.

Take this prescription to your druggist and get him to put it up for you.

It will keep for years. Take it home and put it away in your medicine chest, as described on page 32. Have it marked plainly on the label, "For Croup. Dose: Teaspoonful every half hour till relief, then prolong the intervals as the case may require." Now commence treatment promptly. Give a dose of the above medicine, then make a poultice of bran, add some ground mustard to the poultice, apply it to the breast and throat and keep it there till it reddens the skin. Place the child's feet in hot water, as hot as it can bear it, and keep them there all the while by adding more hot water occasionally till the child gets better and breathes easier. The author has saved the lives of hundreds of children by this prompt treatment. It will not fail if taken in time. But you must keep calm and do not get frightened, so that you do not know what you are doing, and you will be astonished to see how soon your child will come out of those alarming symptoms, and get well quick.

CHILDREN'S CONVULSIONS OR FITS.

These conditions arise from many causes. Sometimes from teething, from worms, or from hard, indigestible food that has been eaten—anything that will tend to irritate the stomach and bowels; or the overloading of the stomach may produce those convulsions. There may be something wrong with the brain, or they may be produced from previous injury, from a fall, or in some other way. But if the child is suffering from a fit, do not get frightened or excited; but take things calmly, for you can work faster when you are cool and deliberate, and to a good deal better advantage, by collecting your thoughts and working by the dictates of your deliberate judgment. *First,* seek at once the advice of your physician. If he is not at hand when the fit comes on take some cloths and dip them into some hot mustard water and wrap up the child's feet and lower parts of the limbs till the skin is quite red, and as soon as opportunity is offered give a teaspoonful of syrup of ipecac, or 20 drops of tincture of lobelia, (each of which should always be kept in your medicine chest, see page 32), and try to induce sickness at the stomach and vomiting, if possible. If the head should appear hot you should apply cold water. This is good treatment and often will bring the child out all right. But when the doctor comes he will find out the cause, and prescribe for you accordingly.

DIARRHŒA.

Bowel complaint occurs every Summer, and often proves fatal to young children. It has been thought the eating of fruits was the cause of children's diarrhœa, as it generally occurs at the time that the fruits are ripening and being gathered. But we think that good, ripe fruit, if perfectly sound and fresh, will do no harm in most cases. While we believe that half-ripe or decayed fruits or vegetables are very unhealthy and but little better than poison. Now, it requires very good judgment to manage successfully all diseases of this kind, and no person, ignorant of medicine, should ever tamper with the life of a child by experiment. Neither should they delay, with the hope of the child getting well of itself. Delays and ignorance in the management of such diseases have been the cause of many deaths. In many cases, where it is allowed to run too long, there are generally very serious complications set up that cannot be very easily controlled. But it is your duty to commence at once with the proper food and the simple remedies, such as described on pages 21, 24 and 25. This will do no harm, and in many cases will cure the case in two or three days. But if there is no change in that time, you should consult your physician at once, who will tell you, if he is an intelligent physician, that you have given the patient the right treatment, and he will not order you to change the diet.

DYSENTERY OR BLOODY FLUX.

This distressing disease, of all others, may be controlled and cured by very simple methods, if not let run too long, till it becomes chronic. The first thing to be done, as in Diarrhœa, is to stop all kinds of food, except the beef extract, milk punch, oatmeal water and mush, as described on pages 14, 15, 16 and 17. But slippery elm, or flax-seed teas made from the water, or from the oatmeal, used as injections after each evacuation from the bowels, are not to be *omitted*. About two tablespoonfuls at a time, or as much as can be retained for a while. Bilious persons, having the obstinate form of this disease, will find great virtue in the following prescription:

Turkey rhubarb and willow charcoal, of each (pulverized) one tablespoonful.

Of saleratus, a piece as large as a hazel-nut.

(The charcoal, put up in bottles, can be had at the drug store.)

The golden seal (hydrastis) half a teaspoonful.

Add these ingredients to a tumblerful of water; stir up well; let it stand covered up twelve hours, when, after thoroughly stirring it, the liquid will be ready for use.

Dose: Teaspoonful of the liquid once in every four hours during the day.

Now then, remember that you are never to wake up at night to take medicine. Sleep will do you more good than to be disturbed of a quiet, easy sleep. We cannot too strongly urge the value of *hand magnetism*. In restoring the balance of health to the system, not only in this but in every disease, no matter what, and especially would we impress upon you to remember that in all stomach and bowel troubles, the *Will* is a very powerful physician. Therefore, do not fail to avail yourself of his skill and beneficence. Always keep your feet and bowels warm and dry. Always sleep with your mouth closed, that the air may pass up through the nostrils into your lungs, that it may be pure and more *magnetic*, and therefore more energizing to your system, and thank the Universal God of Nature that in Him you "live and move and have a being," and your face will soon shine with gladness, and your cheeks will blush with intensified vigor.

Medicines for a Happy Home.

Not only should we cultivate such tempers as serve to render the intercourse of home amiable and affectionate, but we should strive to adorn it with those charms which good sense, judgment and refinement that is so easily imparted to it. We say, easily, for there are persons who think that a home cannot be made beautiful without a considerable outlay of expense in money. Such people are in great error. It costs but very little to have a neat flower-garden, and to surround your dwelling with those simple beauties which delight the eye far more than expensive objects. Nature delights in beauty; she loves to brighten the landscape and make it agreeable to the eye. She hangs the ivy all around the ruin, as well as runs it over the stumps of withered trees. She twines the graceful vine. A thousand arts she practices to animate and please the mind. Follow her example, and do for yourself what she is always laboring to do for you.—*Cotton*.

We are glad to make the above quotation, for it is not only a medical whisper, but rather a short sermon on love, which may prove the best remedy after all to heal many of the infirmities; the best medicine in our pharmacy that we have got, for perhaps you have lost the bright, fresh feelings of the soul.

But we would add, if the writer had only made a more comprehensive supposition (including all the married throughout the world), we could reply affirmatively; except, of course, all of such ordinary broils—those which are always so indispensable as to meet the demands of honest hunger. Let the already truly married still keep up the practice of early courtship. Don't let the principles of Harmonial Love and wisdom ever become old and stale, and die out of your hearts, for it will always sound sweet to be again and again told that we are loved and appreciated by our conjugal companion; for it always acts upon the soul like a tonic. No matter how tired and vexed and worn out with the duties of the day, it will always stimulate you to new strength and vigor. And let all those who are about to embark upon their conjugal existence, regulate all of their attachments, and live by spiritual delicacy and private truthfulness. Now, if all those who chance to read this prescription, will try it, we feel that we could guarantee that such a house would be a natural sanctuary of heavenly blessedness. The family circle would shine and sparkle like a ring of diamonds. Then each throbbing heart would be a wellspring of love, tenderness, grace and gladness. All good angels would go in and out of such a sunny home, just exactly as the healthy children thereof would glide to and fro on the swift feet of unrestrained enjoyment.

A divine joy is certain to pavilion such a happy home, and one tender hand is sure to embrace all hearts which come within its influence, for it would be the very Gates of Heaven.

Motherhood.

This is a question which nearly all writers have evaded as harsh, untimely, or felt that it would not be accepted as modest; but we feel that the time has come when all people should put away all such false modesty, and deal with the real facts as they are, and such important facts that we all should want to know, and we all must meet them sooner or later, whether we will or not.

Motherhood is the crowning glory of Womanhood. But the ambition of the mother should be that of bringing of the germ of able-bodied, great-hearted, glorious men and women, who will always be ready to do and to dare for the truth's sake, for humanity's sake. The salvation of the human race all lies in the practical recognition of one important principle—one which, by future generations, if not now, in the light of our present science, must be pre-eminently acknowledged as an unquestionable truth, viz: That she, who is the continued originator of the race, she, whose power and influence for weal or woe, must be handed down through her posterity during all coming time, she must be educated to, and shall be granted the inalienable, indisputable right to determine for herself when she can lovingly take upon herself the responsibilities of Motherhood. The time has already come when the mass of our thinking people have come to see and to know the one important, but hitherto neglected, lesson learnt, that we are guilty of a heinous crime, and one which nature never pardons, when we will knowingly allow ourselves to become the instruments of bringing into existence human beings whose lives are a curse to the world and to themselves, rather than a blessing. Young men as well as old must also be educated up to this point, to see the facts as they really are.

Till within a very short period physiology has formed no part of the education of parents, and the simplest elements of anatomy have been entirely unknown to mothers; Maidens have entered upon the possibilities of maternity without the slightest information regarding the structure of their bodies, and still less of the powers of fœtal development and intelligent understanding of the inevitable inquiries attending its arrest; and what is still more ludicrous, were it not so very sad, ignorant even of the conditions of parturition. This, we claim, is all wrong; besides there is no excuse for it. We must charge it upon an ignorant Father or Motherhood—Motherhood not yet conscious of its high duties, to instruct their children, at least as far as they know themselves, as well as to urge it upon their children to seek for all the knowledge upon those subjects that they can possibly avail themselves of.

It must be clear to every thinking mind, that it is not probable that there will be any visible decrease in the crime of this world till the pulpit and the press, as well as the law-making power, are convinced that no persuasion, or education, or even punishment, or statutory enactments, can ever be made to cure those who are organically, morally, mentally or physically diseased. As the unborn individual cannot be consulted as to the character of his mind, or his intellectual powers, he is, therefore, dependent upon the condition, and the character, and the intellectual and moral character of his immediate progenitors. Indeed, he has no more control over his moral or mental organization than he has over the color of his eyes or his hair.

Our organization is *made for us and not by us.* Our present educational and religious institutions have not, and cannot, *prevent* the commission or increase of crime.

Why has not man sought out the means of developing and perfecting the human forms of his children as well as he has improved the stock of the animal kingdom below him? We do not want passionless men, but men with strong passion, held resolutely under the check of an enlightened reason and conscientious individualty. It is high time that marriage should be regarded as something higher and nobler than a mere condition granting license to the passions. Let human beings enter into the marriage relation for the sole purpose of companionship, for mutual improvement, and· for the development of their own and each other's noblest, best traits of character. Then, when offspring is desired, let the prospective father and mother seek to combine the very best advantages for the expression of their own and each other's forces, so that their children shall enter upon their earthly career with all of those excellencies of physique and character that adorn the noblest specimens of man or womanhood. The children of such parents, conceived under such conditions, receive, at the moment of conception, an impetus towards the good and the imperishable that no vicissitudes of life can ever obliterate. Such children will never fall into vice, but rather, as we see them grow up to maturity, the very sight of such noble specimens of men and women will be looked upon and considered as the protecting arms thrown out and around to embrace and protect the human race. Happy are the parents whose children love life and all of its opportunities. Happy are the children whose parents derive the greatest joy from their beautiful lives.

Maxims.

1st. Never eat a late supper and go to bed with a full stomach.

2d. Never sleep with your hands over your head. It impedes the circulation, and will produce heart disease.

3d. Never bathe the head with *cold water*, but hot, for all diseases of the brain.

4th. Human magnetism, the life principle, may be imparted from one to another, and is a very potent medicine in all diseases.

5th. Sorrow, grief, fear or any other extraordinary emotion, *will cause disease*. So to be well you must be cheerful and wear a pleasant countenance.

6th. Never allow a child to sleep with an adult. There is an invisible magnetic atmosphere of sympathy emanating from and subsisting between individuals, which, if youth and maturity is brought into close conjunction, will always result in permanent injury to the youngest organization. It is a well ascertained fact that the *aged* will attract vigor and youthfulness from the young, therefore disease will always draw strength from the healthy, should the two continue to sleep together.

7th. Never sleep upon any description of *feathers*, for they impart no life-giving element; but will always draw from you many of the atmospherical energies which emenate from and surround you at all times, and you will always arise in the morning tired and weary, without knowing that it was the feathers which had exhausted all of your vital strength.

8th. Never permit a sick and feverish person to wear the same garment, or repose between the same sheets, longer than two days, because the positive disease of the patient, during the fever, is always absorbed by the contagious substances of the body.

9th. You should never frighten, deceive or tell a lie to your child, because it is so unnatural, and besides it is very wicked.

10th. Never love your child unrighteously. That is to say, never permit your love to smother your judgment nor blind the voice of reason, for you must know that sympathy (or love) is only serviceable when wisely bestowed.

11th. It is more easy to manage and educate a child before its birth than it ever will be subsequent to that event, because the individualism is moulded, and consequently manufactured, more or less perfect in the native womb, and because, also, birth is before thinking.

12th. Never make your child feel you to be its master, nor an inferior, nor a superior, but an honorable associate. You should always substitute examples, truth and association for deception and lies, in your so-called family government.

13th. You must learn to *will* and act, ere the child comes to live among you, as you would have the child will and act before the world.

14th. The unborn child is a mirror, which will faithfully reflect all the wickedness and imperfections, or the goodness or righteousness, of its immediate progenitors. The era is nigh when even all the hidden vices, as well as the secret transgressions of both the ignorant and educated parents will be recognized and read in the face, form and character of their offspring.—*Davis.*

15th. Learn your child to do your will, and never decide without just foundation; or, should you hastily decide, never alter your decision without first explaining, to the comprehension of your child, your reason or reasons for so doing. But it is far better to have your child have perfect confidence in your wisdom.

Cause and Cure of Female Weakness.

What means these peace-destroying symptoms? Bearing down in the lower part of the abdomen, heat, dull pain, burning, weakness in the small of the back, sore place on the spine, small of the back so tender to the touch, dragging, aching in the loins, indisposition to bodily exercise, dread of walking—either far or fast, the feeling wearied and then of numbness in the limbs. Why are our married women so capricious of temper, so childish, at times so given to transition from cold sensations to that of hot flashes; then from amiableness to peevishness, and fretful, with scrofulous swellings? Why are our children born with broken-down blood globules floating through their infant hearts? Why do their young bones absolutely ache with voluptious fatigue, transmitted by ignorant parents?

Every ganglionic center is a telegraphic station; it receives impressions and transmits the signs and disturbances from point to point. Who wonders that our children are scrofulous, and so fond of sweets and stimulants? Who, that can trace the relation between one cause and another, will still grope around yet longer and ask the learned physician to explain why women are sick and unfit for ordinary duties of house-keeping? The principal cause of woman's suffering lies in Prolapsus Uteri, (falling of the womb,) Retroversions, Antiversion, and all other kinds of displacement; Whites, (Leucorrhea,) then inflammation and ulceration of the womb. Those are the main causes which afflict three-fourths of the women of this country; yes, it is no use to attempt to disguise the fact that they are suffering, eking out a miserable existence, many of them without hope that there is any relief to be found for them, while many others, through false modesty, suffer and die in silence rather than consult a competent physician for relief; but, nevertheless, sooner or later the truth must be told that the main CAUSE of all of these reproductive diseases are caused originally by excessive and *unrestrained* indulgences of the animal inclinations, through ignorance. Neither man nor woman have comprehended the primal cause of their suffering; or what would be still worse—those, who knowing the truth, will further practice the ungodly habit of intemperate reproduction. But, if you would be wise and strong, you should seek advice from intelligent persons, and reading books upon these subjects. Fathers and mothers should commence the teaching of their children, as early in life as they could understand, all that they know themselves, as well as to surround them with useful books to read, that their children should not grow up in ignorance of the natural laws and functions of the organs of the human body, and their uses, as well as to know the consequent suffering from their abuses. This subject is entirely too broad and deep for us to go into full details. This little book is intended only to hint at the different subjects and point out the way you should do, and give you such knowledge and treatment that is practicable, which will tend to relieve your immediate suffering, as well as to teach you how you can keep well, and to prevent the suffering of others.

But, first of all, we must give you our opinion, based upon twenty years' practice with female diseases, that the introductions and use of all kinds of Pessaries and Uterine Supporters have proved a failure to cure the falling of the womb. They are not only useless, but they have proved to be very injurious. Now, the treatment we propose to give you is very simple, but *radical* and *positive*. Every woman suffering from those diseases should provide herself with a good soft rubber syringe—a No. 1 Davis or Mattson's are the best. With this instrument, properly used, she can cure herself of Whites, (Leucorrhea,) and many other kinds of vaginal irritations.

REMEDY No. 1.—Take the white of one egg, beat it up well on a plate; after which add a tablespoonfull of strained honey, thoroughly amalgamated; after which add it to one pint of blood-warm water, then it is ready for use.

No. 2.—To one pint of blood-warm water add five to six drops of *diluted* sulphuric acid; mix well; ready for use.

No. 3.—One pint of warm water, one teaspoonful of baking soda added; dissolve and mix well; ready for use.

No. 4.—One quart of warm water; add one teaspoonfull of table-salt; dissolve well; ready for use.

No. 5.—One pint of warm water; add tablespoonful of ox-gall; mix; ready for use.

Nos. 6 and 7.—Make a decoction from the plantain leaves, which grow in your door-yards in great abundance, or a decoction from the walnut leaves, and use a quart at one time, blood warm.

DIRECTIONS FOR USING THE SAME.—Where there is much discharge from the vagina, you should first cleanse the part out with castile soap-suds, injected with your syringe; after which you can use Remedy No. 1, commencing in the morning and inject slowly, that the medicine may have a chance to affect all the parts of the vagina. At noon you can use No. 2, and at bedtime use No. 3 in like manner. Use those remedies for several days in succession, then you can substitute either one of the other remedies, and thus you can alternate them until you get well. In the meantime you can take the following medicine internally; get your druggist to put it up:

      Fluid extract black cohosh......................1 drachm.
      Fluid extract chamomile........................   "
      Fluid extract of dandelion ....1 ounce.
      Glycerine sufficient to make a four-ounce mixture.
      DOSE.—Teaspoonfull one hour after each meal.

This treatment persisted in will cure any ordinary case.

In cases of falling of the womb, or where there is a little inflammation or ulceration, it can be cured by the following medicine; get your druggist to put it up for you:

Glycerine..6 ounces.
Tanic acid..½ "

Mix by a gentle heat till the acid is all dissolved. Then take a tuft of fine cotton, about the size of a small hulled walnut; after tucking the fringed edges over to the center, take four stitches through the tuft of cotton with a strong patent thread; soak this tuft of cotton in the glycerine and tannin medicine. Just before going to bed, let some lady friend insert this tuft of cotton (soaked with glycerine of tannin) up the vagina as far as she can push it with the finger, leaving three or four inches of the thread hanging outside; keep this in till ten or eleven o'clock next day, then by the thread you can draw it out and throw it away; then inject a little warm soap-suds, and rinse out the parts. This tanic acid mixture will stain your sheets or clothes; better prepare for it. This treatment, with the cotton tuft and glycerine medicine, can be kept up every evening, or every other day, or third day, as the nature of the case demands; from five to six applications is generally sufficient to effect a cure, by keeping up the other washes and injections between times.

This method of treatment and handling those diseases are simple and harmless, and perfectly reliable. The author has had no occasion to use any other remedies for many years. The treatment is always followed with marked success. However, we might add, that when there is much irritation, smarting or burning sensation in the walls of the vagina, it can soon be healed up and cured, by beating up well on a dinner plate, the white of one egg, and add it to a pint of warm water, to be used with the syringe as an injection-wash, in place of one of the other injections.

Accidents and Emergencies.

Under this head, which properly commences on page 33, we will continue here by giving you a number of prescriptions.

BURNS AND SCALDS.

1. A liniment composed of equal parts of lime-water and linseed oil, is a superior application for burns. The lime-water alone is excellent.

2. Dissolve two ounces of alum in one pint of hot water. Saturate cotton cloths with this solution and keep the burn well wrapped in them. The pain will quickly cease and the process of healing will soon commence.

3. Two tablespoonfuls of bicarbonate of soda dissolved in one pint of hot water. Saturate cotton cloths with this solution and keep the parts well wrapped up, and the cloths constantly kept wet with this solution. The pain will soon cease and the process of healing will soon commence.

Care should be taken not to let the parts be exposed to the air for one moment from the time of the first application, by the change of the dressing. This can be accomplished by handling the burnt parts under the water while dressing. Burns and scalds will heal rapidly, without leaving a scar, if attended to in this manner.

When the clothing of a person catches fire, throw them on the ground and roll them up in a piece of carpet, or a bed quilt is still better. This will extinguish the flames. If those articles are not at hand then take your coat and use it instead. Begin the wrapping at the neck and shoulders and wrap downwards, so as to keep the flames from the head and face. Cover all again with damp clothes, several thicknesses. This will soon extinguish the flames; after which the burnt parts can be dressed with Cosmoline. This is a new remedy, and it is an excellent one. After covering the Cosmoline with only one thickness of cotton cloth, then wrap the entire dressing with raw cotton to exclude the air. If the weather is very warm the Cosmoline dressing should be renewed twice per day; otherwise, every other day will be sufficient. The dressing should take place under the water, if possible, to exclude the air from the burnt parts.

The above remedies and treatment are the best *known*, and adopted by all the profession. We present quite a number of them, from the fact that it often happens that only one remedy is at hand and ready for use, whilst the others might not be had without the loss of much valuable time, while any one of the above is very good.

POISON VINE; POISON OAK.

REMEDY.—Mix a small quantity of starch with sufficient glycerine to form a thick paste and apply to the poisoned parts. This is excellent. One application is generally sufficient to effect a cure; if not, it may be repeated on the following morning. This, in the author's hands, has never been known to fail. Before the application, bathe the parts in hot water, almost hot enough to scald the flesh.

But, as this remedy may not always be at hand, we will give another:

Baking soda, or common washing soda, will remove this difficulty very promptly by adding sufficient water to the soda to form a paste, and apply it thoroughly once or twice a day. It will usually kill the poison in from two to four days.

The following is from Prof. Bundy, of Oakland, Cal., in which State poisoning is of very frequent occurrence from the poison oak. Take of the

    Fluid extract of grindelia robusta............2 drachms.
    Glycerine....................................2 ounces.

Mix and apply to the affected parts three or four times daily.

This is a new remedy, and is a specific for the poison oak poisoning; in fact so much so that no other treatment need be mentioned. This remedy can now be always found at the drug stores.

SPIDER BITES.

1. Catnip and plantain (which grows in nearly everybody's dooryard) equal parts, bruised and applied to the wound, is a prompt and effectual remedy for the cure of the bite of a spider, or any other insect. A teaspoonful of the juice of the plantain should be taken internally every hour, at the same time. This is also a cure for a hornet or a bee sting. Then in case these remedies are not handy we will give you some other remedies.

2. Table salt and baking power, equal parts, bound on the parts. This will immediately arrest the swelling and relieve the pain.

3. The common onion is another remedy for the same purpose. A piece is to be cut off and at once applied on the wound. Dr. Hill uses no other remedy than this for stings, etc. If the pieces of onion are changed every few minutes, the pain, he says, diminishes immediately.

ACCESSORY MEASURES.—If a wasp, or other stinging insect, be the cause of the trouble, examination must be made to see if the sting is left in the flesh, as this is often the case. Then the sting must be extracted by the fingers or a pair of fine-pointed forceps.

SNAKE BITES.

The first object to be attempted, in such cases, is to arrest the circulation of the blood, from the part bitten, as soon as possible. This can be done by tying a handkerchief or rope tightly around the limb, between the wound and the heart, as directed on page 33 (to stop hemorrhage.) The wound should be sucked with all the force the patient can command, or have some person do it for him. No danger attached to the person thus sucking the wound, so long as the poison does not come in contact with any abraded or raw surface of the mouth or other parts of the body. If any considerable time has elapsed after the bite, and before the application has been made, then there should be made a small incision of the flesh, with a knife, across the wound, in order, more readily, to admit the solution into the wound, after which the bruised plantain will do you good service, as before described. If that is not at hand, the next best remedy is moistened saleratus and bound on the bite. Then dissolve more and keep the parts wet with it for a few hours. This remedy has not yet been known to fail to cure the bite of a snake.

The old remedy is to drink plenty of good brandy till you get intoxicated; and then it sometimes fails.

We would rather use the plaintain externally and internally.

CRAMP IN THE PIT OF THE STOMACH.

Severe, pinching, gnawing, or contractive pains in the stomach, generally occurring after taking food.

CAUSE.—Highly seasoned or indigestible food; stimulants, coffee and tobacco; long fasting, exposure to cold or damp, etc. It is usually but a symptom of indigestion.

REMEDY.—Most forms of this difficulty can be effectually cured in a few minutes by a very simple means:

Take a teacupful of hot water, and add to it a heaping tablespoonful of sugar. Drink it down slowly, as hot as possible. In some cases it may be necessary to repeat the dose in twenty or thirty minutes; but it is seldom that more than one dose will be needed.

Another means is to place a mustard poultice on the stomach and allow it to remain till considerable redness is produced; then follow this with a hot fomentation of hops or tansy. If this should occur in the middle of the night, the patient should apply friction over the stomach. This rubbing with the hand, with an active *will*, until considerable redness, with a high degree of heat, is produced. It alone will often afford effectual relief. However, the patient subject to these attacks should shun all articles of food which excite attacks of this disease, and live on plain, easily digested food, spend his time in the fresh air and sunlight, and take regular active exercise.

BILIOUS COLIC OR CRAMP COLIC.

Many persons are subject to this distressing disease and suffer for hours without obtaining relief, when it is the simplest thing to cure in the world.

Take of the fluid extract of (diascora villosa) wild yam, 30 drops in about one swallow of hot water, at a dose; repeat it in 30 minutes if necessary. In the meantime take one pint of warm water, add half teaspoonful of salt to it, stir till dissolved, and inject it slowly into the bowels with a syringe. Retain it as long as possible. This will evacuate the bowels in less than 30 minutes, and you will get prompt relief.

JAUNDICE.

The fringe-tree (chionanthus)—"Old Man's Gray Beard," as it is sometimes called. This is a new remedy for this disease, introduced to the profession by Prof. B. J. M. Goss. He says it is a specific for jaundice. This article can be procured at the drug store. Call for the fluid extract. The dose is a teaspoonful, in a little sweetened water, before each meal. In ten days your jaundice is all gone.

However, the jaundice may be complicated with other diseases. In this case, after your trial, you can consult your physician.

NEURALGIA.

It is very important for those who are afflicted with this distressing disease to be prepared with a few remedies at hand, and with their judicious use they need not suffer very long with this distressing disease.

REMEDY 1.—Take half a teaspoonful of sal amonia and four tablespoonfuls of camphor-water; mix.

Dose: Teaspoonful, and repeat several times at intervals of ten minutes, if the pain be not relieved at once, as many neuralgia patients can attest.

Camphor-water may be prepared by adding one teaspoonful of the strong spirits of camphor to half teacupful of water. But one remedy will hardly ever cure every case of this disease.

There is a new remedy discovered, and one that is reported by the profession to be of superior efficacy in the cure of neuralgia; in fact it is regarded as an effectual cure in this disease. It is the sulphate of nickel. Have your druggist prepare it for you by rubbing one grain of it in a mortar with nine grains of sugar of milk; triturate well. Divide it into two-grain doses. One dose is often sufficient to relieve the severest paroxysm of pain. If it should not do so, the dose can be repeated every one or two hours until the pain ceases. Prof. Hale, of Chicago, has reported many very grave cases of neuralgia cured by this remedy. The author has used it in several very old cases of neuralgia, and has been utterly astonished to see how prompt this remedy relieved that most excruciating malady, especially if it is of a periodical character.

It is useless to treat this disease with liniments. Fomentations are much better than all the pain-killers in America.

The hot air sweat, repeated several times, is the most reliable permanent cure that we know of. (See description of Bath.)

EARACHE.

First, the ear should be carefully examined to see if any foreign substance is in it, that may provoke the difficulty, the removal of which will relieve at once. If nothing of the kind is discovered, we may know it to be the result of a cold. Then proceed as follows:

Heat a brick or stone and wrap it up with a damp cloth or towel, and place to the ear, heating and sweating it freely. At the same time take equal parts of sweet oil and glycerine, teaspoonful each, and add 10 drops of laudanum to this; mix well by warming it over the stove. Then take a straw or little stick, from the end of which drop 3 or 4 drops of this mixture into the ear. This will give you prompt relief at once.

DIPHTHERIA.

Diphtheria is scarcely more than a modification of scarlet fever. The patient first complains of lassitude, aches all over, especially in the back and hips, head aches, loss of appetite, rigors and chills, active and quick pulse, a light-furred tongue, redness in the back of the mouth, enlargement of the glands about the neck, a hot, dry skin, and in most cases an exudation formed upon the mucous surfaces of the upper air passages. This soon becomes organized into a tough, white membrane, covering the soft palate and tonsils. These sometimes degenerate into ulcers. The breathing, in consequence of the condition of the membranes and air passages, becomes hurried and labored, and the patient becomes very restless and uneasy, pulse quick and frequent, the asphyxia ensuing ends in death. The breath becomes fœted. No one, after breathing the breath and exudations arising from a diphtheric patient, can ever mistake this disease. It generally rages as an epidemic, and is regarded as contagious.

TREATMENT.—The first step in the treatment should be an emetic by a copious draught of milk-warm water with a little salt and ground mustard added to the warm water. This should be drank slowly and continuedly until the patient vomits. No danger, don't be afraid of too much water; it is harmless. The vomiting will, at the same time, produce free perspiration, which is highly necessary, and should be kept up by the use of the tincture of gelseminum and aconite root, of each 20 drops, added to a half-tumbler of water.

Dose: Teaspoonful every hour.

The kidneys should be kept in vigorous operation. Flannel cloths should be wet with the compound tincture of capsicum, myrrh and lobelia, and should be changed every half hour, and applied as hot as the patient can bear it, till the disease is under control, taking care that the throat is well protected from the cold air after the hot flannel cloths are abandoned. The patient should be kept in bed with hot jugs kept to the feet, and a gentle perspiration should be kept up. The bowels should be evacuated by injections of warm water.

The following prescription the author has found to be a specific to kill the ulcers and exudations that gather upon the tonsils and mucous membranes in the throat:

Chlorate of potassium	1 drachm.
Fluid extract wild yam (diascora villosa)	½ drachm.
Hydrate of chloral	1 drachm.
Tincture of muriate of iron	1 drachm.
Carbolic acid	5 drops.
Glycerine	3 ounces.

Mix well.

You can get your druggist to put this prescription up for you. Now, with a camel-hair brush you can touch the tonsils and all the exudations in the throat three or four times per day with this medicine. If the patient swallows a little it will do no harm. If the medicine appears to be a little too strong, it can be reduced with a little water. You will be astonished to see how soon the ulcers will clean off and begin to heal up under this treatment.

Give the patient plenty of milk punch, (see page 17, how to make it.) Add plenty of brandy, as it is said, by late observers, that good whisky or brandy is a prophylactic in diphtheria. Hence you can add more than usual to the milk punch. Also give the extract of beef, (see page 14). In convalescing, the patient should have a good sponge bath every day, followed by a brisk rubbing with the bare hands by the nurse or some genial friend.

ERYSIPELAS (ST. ANTHONY'S FIRE.)

CAUSE—Exposure to cold; impaired digestion; wounds; particularly from dissecting and surgical instruments; badly ventilated and over-crowded apartments; certain condition of the atmosphere and a morbid state of the blood from disease; the habitual use of stimulants, etc., and consequently debility. The tendency of the disease is to attack different parts of the body simultaneously, which furnishes us with evidence of its origin in a bad condition of the blood. The chief existing cause of Erysipelas is a recent wound, and the predisposing cause is inattention to the laws of health, combined, perhaps, with a personal or family tendency to the disease. Erysipelas is known by its inflammatory redness of the skin, and its rapid tendency of spreading over the body, with considerable puffy swelling, tenderness, painful burning, tingling and tension. The color varies from a faint-red to a dark-red or purplish color, becoming white under pressure but returning to its former color on the removal of the pressure. An attack is usually ushered in with shivering, languor, headache and nausea; bilious vomiting with the ordinary symptoms of inflammatory fever, accompanied or followed by inflammation of the parts affected. When erysipelas attacks the face, it nearly always commences at the side of the nose near the angle of the eye.

REMEDIES AND TREATMENT. —Applications, externally used, should always be put on warm, whatever form the disease may assume; cold applications should never be made, as they interfere with the free circulation of the blood, and the nutrition of the part; and they always increase rather than diminish the extent of the severity of the disease.

There are many kinds of treatment for this disease, but we will endeavor to give you only that which has been adopted by the author, which, in every case, has proved to be the most successful and can be relied upon.

A poultice made from the cranberries, stewed and cooked in the usual way, and applied blood-warm, is a very valuable remedy for outward application. If those are out of season, the next best remedy is a decoction of strong tea made from the inner bark of the burr-oak tree, and use this to make a bread poultice, and apply it. If this cannot be had, the next best is sulphite of soda, half an ounce, to a pint of blood-warm rain-water; dissolve well. A cotton cloth wet well in this and laid over the affected parts, one thickness, and kept wet by often changing. However, the cloth should be thoroughly washed in clean water before putting it in the soda medicine.

Again: Also the hamamelis, the witch-hazel, as it is sometimes called, used in the same way as the soda solution; but use it full strength.

Also, I have used a gill of good brandy with the juice of 2 lemons added. Keep the affected parts well moistened with either of those remedies till the inflammation is well subdued. We have always been successful with those remedies used in this way. Sometimes we alternate with two of those remedies, first using one, then the other, until the inflammatory action is entirely under control.

But this disease must be taken in time. It will not do to postpone the treatment for one moment, as the disease is a very dangerous one.

For the internal treatment we use the following prescription:

Muriate tincture of iron .... 3 drachms.
Diluted carbolic acid .... $\frac{1}{2}$ drachm.
Fluid ext. wild indigo (baptisia tinctoria) 1 drachm.
Glycerine sufficient to make a four ounce mixture.

Dose: Teaspoonful every two hours.

If it is of the facial erysipelas with much fever, it must be controlled by the mother tincture of belladonna and aconite. They can be procured at the homeopathic pharmacy. Give 10 drops of each in a half-tumbler of water; mix well.

Dose: Teaspoonful every hour if the fever is high, and the iron mixture every three hours, till the fever is controlled; then stop and give the first tincture of iron medicine every two hours.

Keep the bowels open by injections of salt and water, as described in other pages of this book. This treatment will do you good service in this disease.

SCARLET FEVER.

Children are far more liable to contract this disease than adults, as very few of the latter ever have this disease, even when exposed. The interval between the exposure and the attack varies from two to five days to three weeks, and patients are known to have the disease without exposure, when it is prevailing in the neighborhood.

GENERAL SYMPTOMS.—Scarlet fever usually commences very suddenly, with the ordinary forerunners of fever, chills, and shivering, succeeded by hot skin, nausea, sometimes vomiting, with rapid pulse, thirst, frontal headache, and sore throat. The last named symptom, sore throat, is generally the earliest complained of by the patient. In about forty-eight hours after the occurrence of those symptoms, the characteristic rash is perceptible, first on the breast, from whence it generally extends and spreads all over the body. These eruptions are bright-red points or spots, which have been compared, by some writers, to look like that of a boiled lobster shell.

These spots either run together and diffuse themselves uniformly over the skin, or else appear in large, irregular patches on different parts of the body. The color of the skin disappears on pressure, but returns on its removal. The appearance of the tongue is characteristic: it is first coated, but the tips and edges are red; the pimples are red and somewhat raised; afterward the tongue cleans off and looks very red and raw. A diffused redness, sometimes of a dark scarlet color, covers the mouth, etc., which all disappears as the febrile symptoms and rash subside. About the fifth day the rash begins to decline, and entirely disappears about the eighth or ninth day, leaving the patient in a very weak condition. The subsequent process of peeling of the cuticle is varied in its duration; it takes place in the form of scurf, from the face and trunk, but from the hands and feet large flakes are separated, sometimes coming away entire like a glove or slipper.

This also is a very dangerous disease, and should have prompt attention. We shall advise you to send for your physician, as this disease is apt to be followed by serious complications, and not attempt treatment yourself. But, as the external treatment is the most essential to be attended to, the author will give you that which we always employ, no matter what the complications are, and it is always called for in every case, and your family physician, if he is an intelligent one, will not object to it, as it will not interfere with his internal treatment. As this is a cutaneous disease, the battle-ground to be fought is upon the surface; hence we should advise you by all means to give a warm sponge bath every night, followed by greasing the entire body all over with an uncooked fat piece of bacon—in severe cases we always bind thin slices of it upon the neck, breast and soles of the feet. We shall urge this treatment upon you, as it is always called for and highly effectual. If attended to promptly it will never fail to cure the patient with but little other treatment.

SMALLPOX (Variola).

This disease is too well known to need a particular description. It is always caused or communicated by contagion; that is, caught from others who have it. There are two forms of this disease—the Confluent, when the vesicles are so thick that they run together; and the Distinct, when they are separate. Then we have Varioloid, or Smallpox modified by constitutional predisposition—we won't say by vaccination, because we don't believe that vaccination ever prevented a case of smallpox in this world; but, on the contrary, we do know of many cases of confluent smallpox after the patients informed us that they had been vaccinated and that it took well. Therefore we would advise you never to allow your children to be vaccinated under any consideration. Of our own observation of the condition of the human family, which we have formed after an experience of over twenty years in the practice of medicine, we have long since arrived at the conclusion that the inhuman practice of vaccination has caused more deaths than the disease of smallpox ever did, to say nothing of the consumption and scrofulistic wrecks that the sin of vaccination has left all over the world. From conscientious scruples, the author has never yet vaccinated a single individual, and we don't intend to commence now. Our voice shall ever be heard in condemnation of that inhuman practice.

If the rules and laws of health are observed, which we have endeavored to give you in this little book, you need never be any more afraid of smallpox than you need be of any other disease. However, we will proceed to tell you that the treatment in this disease is simple and easy to manage. We have a remedy from London which rivals all others for its simplicity, and, coming as it does so highly recommended, we apprehend that it has accomplished all that is claimed for it:

Dissolve one ounce of cream of tartar in one pint of boiling water. Of this, when cold, give half a gill for the first dose, to an adult. After this is taken, divide the remaining quantity into such doses as, taken three times a day, the whole will last three days.

It is said that this simple remedy has restored thousands of cases, and will effectually cure this disease in five or six days, leaving no pit marks and no blindness, as is sometimes the case when otherwise treated, and always prevents the tedious lingering of convalescence; besides, it can be taken at any time, being preventive as well as curative. The use of it is so effectual that, were it popularly employed, it would dispense with the unnatural law of vaccination and the very costly staff of vaccinators.

Another remedy, more in use in some parts of Europe, and also in China, and said to be the most successful ever employed in those countries, and perfectly effectual, is to apply to the chest an ointment made by combining tartar-emetic and croton-oil with lard. This application should be made when the fever is at its height and just before the eruptions appear. This causes the whole of the eruptions to appear on this part of the body, and thus relieves the internal organs and the face, on which there will be no pitting.

WORMS.

Worm troubles are not so common as generally supposed. Almost every irritation or abnormal condition of a child is attributed by the parents or others to the presence of worms, and the little sufferer is often made worse by the use of medicines. In no case, however, should the child be purged and medicated for worms unless it is quite positive that such are present. Rarely do they exist without some evidence being shown in the discharges from the bowels; hence these should be carefully examined. Large sums of money are annually spent in this way. Get your druggist to put you up the following prescription:

Santonine .... 4 grains.
Sugar of milk .... 10 grains.
Mix and triturate and divide into six powders.

Give one of these powders three times per day for three days; then skip two days; then give the other powders in like manner. Just pour it from the paper into the child's mouth—the medicine is pleasant—after which give the patient a sup of water. The child will not object to it. This the next day is to be followed by a little salt and water. The child's food may contain an extra quantity of salt for a few days, but this excess of salt is to be discontinued when it is rid of the worms. This is all the treatment that any child need have for worms.

CHRONIC SORE EYES.

Chronic sore eyes, or indeed any kind of acute sore eyes, can be cured in the most simple way. We have cured hundreds of cases after trying all other means. We know what we are talking about. Never allow anybody to drop "eye-water" in your eyes—never. Get a clean piece of ice, and after washing a crock or other suitable vessel out clean, let the ice melt in the crock in the sun, after which strain, if there is sediment in it; then bottle this ice water in a clean bottle. This is the purest water that can be had, as the freezing process takes out all inorganic matter. Now, after you have washed your hands and face clean with soap, taking care that no soap gets into the eyes, then rinse the hands and face with clear, fresh water. Now take half a pint of this ice water, poured into a very clean vessel; add less than half a teaspoonful of table salt. After dissolving it, bathe the eyes gently with this water, opening the eyes occasionally so that a little of the salt-water will get into the eyes. Repeat the process three or four times a day. If there is much inflammation, this can be subdued by applying a poultice made from scraping a raw potato and laying it over the eyes, changing it every two hours. This can be alternated with a wet cloth, single thickness, laid over the eyes, wet from the ice water and salt mixture. The author has cured hundreds of cases in this way after all other means had failed. The grand secret in curing sore eyes is to keep your dirty fingers out of your eyes; also, the secretions which are constantly running out of the eyes and down the face, which will naturally get upon the fingers and back into the eyes if you are not careful and keep your hands washed clean when you attempt to treat the eyes. However, if your system is otherwise not in a healthy condition, this will have to be attended to.

SICK HEADACHE.

This distressing disease has received its name from the constant nausea, or sickness of the stomach, which attends the pain in the head.

SYMPTOMS.—This headache is apt to begin in the morning, on waking from a deep sleep, or after sleeping in a closed room, or when some irregularity of diet has been indulged in on the several preceding days. First, there is an oppressive feeling in the head, which gradually increases into a severe pain in the temples or top of the head, followed by a deathly sickness at the stomach, with a sense of tenderness on pressure at the stomach, and sometimes vomiting.

REMEDY.—Now the quickest way to get rid of this most distressing of all sicknes is to empty the stomach at once by an emetic, which can be produced by drinking slowly a large quantity of blood-warm water, with just enough salt added to be tasted. This will wash out and cleanse the stomach at once of all its morbid contents. At the same time you should place your feet in a hot foot-bath; this will induce perspiration, which is highly necessary. Then, as soon as the stomach becomes a little quiet and calm, you can commence the drinking of lemon-water, prepared in the following manner:

Two gills of tepid water, add one teaspoonful of oil or the clear juice of lemon, and drink this quantity every fifteen minutes for one hour. Persons of strong constitutional habits may add more of the juice of the lemon and water at a dose. We have cured hundreds of patients in this simple manner, without a single failure. Often in three hours the patients would be as well as ever they were, and could go about their work as well as usual.

More than one-fourth of the female portion of mankind have experienced sick headache, in a greater or less degree, ever since saleratus was introduced and used as an ingredient in the making of bread and pastries. Therefore, the more nearly it is dispensed with the less of this affection there will be, as well as some other maladies.

However, when there is acidity of the stomach, two teaspoonfuls of pulverized willow charcoal dissolved in a half teacupful of soda water (baking soda will answer) and taken at one dose will cure this form of deranged stomach. There are many other forms of headache arising from other causes too numerous to mention in this little book. Some, however, are from loss of nerve force, or vital force, and some are produced by excess of mental labor or deep sorrow. Those forms of headache are readily cured by the magnetic powers of another person, commonly called Human Magnetism, with which most persons are perfectly familiar. It is done in the following way: First, place the feet of the patient into a hot foot bath, then the operator should stand behind the patient and, with both hands, should make gentle passes from the center of the forehead, and draw the hands gently backward over the top of the head, over the temples and down the spine for a few minutes, then the operator can change his position to the right side of the patient and place the palm of the left hand on the back of the neck, and hold it still in that position, while at the same time he can make gentle passes from the center of the forehead with his right hand down the left side of the face down the left arm to the end of the fingers, then the next pass down over the right side of the face and arm to the end of the fingers of the right side of the patient, and alternate the passes in this way, first down one side then down the other. In thirty minutes you will be astonished to hear your patient declare that his headache has entirely left him.

Human magnetism is a potent agent as an assistant in the cure of all diseases to which the human body is heir, when properly used as such. There are many physicians that are curing disease in this way, at the present day, without the use of a grain of medicine of any kind, and many of them are very successful. The author will give you an essay on the Philosophy of Human Magnetism in the closing chapter of this little book.

CHRONIC RHEUMATISM.

This sometimes follows the acute form of rheumatism, and at othertimes it is a separate and constitutional affection, coming on quite independently of any previous attack. This disease is generally very obstinate, prone to recur, and is often worse at night. In time, the affected limbs lose their power of motion, from the membranes and joints being often affected, the muscles sometimes become permanently contracted and lameness is the result. There is but little fever, no perspiration and less swelling than in acute rheumatism. This form of the disease is often the result of uncured acute forms. It may be limited to one part of the body, or extend to several. It may be fixed or shifting. The author's extended experience in this disease has led us to believe that rheumatism is a disease of the blood. Hence, to expect to cure this disease by the use of liniments, as is usually supposed, is perfectly absurd. However, we often prescribe them as temporary relief till we can have time for the action of other curative remedies. The cause of rheumatism in different individuals is varied. In some persons the cause is from an alkaline condition of the fluids of the body, but in most individuals it is from an acrid condition.

Hence, from this fact the treatment must be varied. In some we give the bicarbonate of soda, 10 grains at a dose, repeated two or three times per day. In others, we give the diluted muriatic acid, half an ounce to five ounces of water; teaspoonful of this in a tumblerful of water, and use it as a drink several times a day. These prescriptions we give you that you can try each till you know which of the two remedies is required in your system. This can be readily told by which of the two remedies is relished the best, for if the system requires the soda it will be desired by the taste more than the acid, and in a few hours it will be followed by marked improvement in the symptoms, and *vice versa*.

At the same time you can be taking the following prescription, which you can get your druggist to put up for you:

<pre>
Fluid extract of black cohosh (cimicifuga
    racemosa) .... 1 drachm.
Fluid ext. poke root (phytolacca decandra) 1 drachm.
Fluid extract of colchicum .... 1 drachm.
Syrup of ginger .... 4 ounces.
</pre>
Mix.

Dose: Teaspoonful every three hours.

For a liniment, for external use, you can use the following:

<pre>
Oil of cedar .... 1 ounce.
Oil of sassafras .... 1 ounce.
Oil of amber .... 1 ounce.
Oil of olive .... 1 ounce.
Hartshorn .... 1 ounce.
Spirits of camphor .... 1 ounce.
Spirits of turpentine .... 1 ounce.
Tincture of laudanum .... 1 ounce.
Tincture of capsicum .... 1 ounce.
Alcohol .... 1 pint.
</pre>
Mix.

Apply twice a day, and keep the parts well wrapped up with flannel.

This treatment, persisted in, together with the alcoholic sweat bath, (as described on page 29, or see cut of both), taken two or three times per week, will cure any ordinary case of rheumatism that we have ever seen.

However, we will give you other prescriptions highly recommended by other authors.

The following is a new remedy that is highly recommended and published as an effectual cure for rheumatism:

"Take the common garden celery, cut it into small pieces and boil it in water until it is soft. Of this liquor let the patient drink freely three or four times per day. To use it as an article of diet prepare it in the following way: Put new milk with a little flour into a sauce-pan with a little nutmeg, and simmer gently, and serve it warm with pieces of toast, and this painful ailment will soon yield."

Such is the declaration of an eminent physician, who has tried it again and again with uniform success.

After this painful disease is broken up it should always be followed with this prescription, as this will act promptly on the kidneys and carry the disease out of the system. It is also good in any kidney trouble; and this is our own prescription:

Fluid extract of Queen of the Meadow
   (eupatorium purpureum).................. one and a half ozs.
Fluid extract of pleurisy root (asclepias tuberosa)... 1 drachm.
Fluid extract of blood root (sanguinaria canadensis)... 10 drops.
Nitrate potass.. 3 drachms.
Glycerine sufficient to make a 4-oz. mixture. Mix.

Dose: Teaspoonful every three hours.

This will take out of your system all the rheumatic poison that is in your blood, after the other remedies are first taken.

SUNSTROKE.

SYMPTOMS.—Most cases are preceded by pain in the head; wandering of thoughts; or an inability to think at all; disturbed vision; irritability of temper; sense of pain or weight at the pit of the stomach; inability to breathe with the usual ease and satisfaction; skin dry and hot, sometimes cold; and very soon the patient feels unable to command his limbs, and finally he sinks down in a state of more or less complete unconsciousness.

REMEDIES.—The old method of applying cold water to the head is bad practice, and should be abandoned.

A better method is to make warm water applications. If hot water cannot be obtained then bathe the head first with tepid water, and, with the hands moistened, rub the neck and whole length of the spine, then the extremities in a downward direction, in order to draw the blood from the brain. As soon as hot water can be obtained, put a dry blanket all around the patient's body. Now wring flannels from the hot water and apply them quickly to the region of the stomach, liver, bowels and spine. Immerse the feet in hot water, or wrap them in hot blankets up as far as the body. Change the flannels and re-wring them from the hot water every eight or ten minutes for half an hour or more. Then remove them as soon as circulation is established, and apply tepid water; then dry well and rub the body briskly with the hands until a glow is produced or perspiration is established. As soon as the patient can swallow, give him hot water to drink and plenty of it, with occasional bits of crushed ice, or a sip of cold water Keep the tepid water on the head all the time changed frequently, and all will be well in a few hours.

PREVENTION.—During the heated term, as it is called, all use of malt, fermented or distilled drinks should be abandoned. Wear a hat that will permit the air to pass through, and have the top lined with one thickness of flannel, or keep a damp silk handkerchief in the crown. Persons who feel the above symptoms must immediately get into the shade and bathe the head in cold water. Everything calculated to impair the strength should be avoided. Sleep is a most wonderful restorer of strength, and the want of it is often caused by a badly assorted late meal of the evening before. Defective ventilation often leads to a condition of affairs favorable to the malady under consideration. Drinking large quantities of ice-cold water, merely because it is cold, particularly before and after meals.

CHOLERA MORBUS.

Cholera Morbus is a violent purging and vomiting, attended with griping in the bowels, with a constant desire to go to stool. It comes on suddenly, and is most common in autumn. There is hardly any disease that kills more quickly than this, when proper means are not used in due time for removing it.

CAUSE.—It is occasioned by a redundancy and putrid acrimony of the bile; food that easily turns sour on the stomach, as butter, fat pork, sweet-meats, pies and cakes, apples or melons, cherries, cucumbers, etc. It sometimes proceeds from poisonous substances taken into the stomach. It may likewise proceed from a violent passion or affection of the mind, such as fear, anger, etc.

SYMPTOMS.—It is generally preceded by heart-burn, sour belching from the stomach and flatulency, with pain in the stomach and intestines. These are followed by excessive vomiting and purging of green, yellow or blackish-colored bile, with distention of the stomach, with violent griping pains. There is likewise great thirst, and often a fixed pain about the region of the navel. Sometimes a cold, clammy sweat. As the disease progresses the pulse sinks so low as to almost become imperceptible, the extremities grow cold, the urine is obstructed and there is palpitation of the heart. Violent hiccoughing, fainting and convulsions are the signs of approaching death.

REMEDY.—Under the head of Recipes and Prescriptions you will find the author's remedy for this disease, and how to use it.

However, we will give one of the old prescriptions, one which, we have no doubt, is very good. But, first, you must keep the surface of your patient warm. Feet and extremities must be wrapped in dry, hot blankets heated by a stove, then hot irons and jugs of hot water kept to the feet and limbs; mustard draft to the stomach till the skin is quite red; and give the following:

Ground black pepper, one tablespoonful.
Table salt, one tablespoonful.
Hot water, half tumblerful.
Cider vinegar, half tumblerful. Mix.

Dose: One teaspoonful every few minutes till the whole is taken.

It is said that this may be relied upon in curing cholera morbus, and also genuine cholera.

First dose may be vomited up; if so, repeat the dose. The vomiting will seldom return.

Stir the medicine well each dose.

CHOLERA INFANTUM.

Sugar of milk	half ounce.
Lactated pepsin	35 grains.
Lactic acid	
Hydrochloric acid	
Aromatic syrup of rhubarb, of each	half drachm.
Tincture of prickly ash berries (xanthoryllum)	1 drachm.
Distilled water	one and a half ozs.
Syrup of lemon	one and a half ozs.

Mix.

Dose. Half teaspoonful every half hour, or hour, as the case may require. If it is too strong for the child, it can be made weak and palatable to suit the judgment.

MEASLES (RUBEOLA).

This disease is a continued infectious fever, preceded by sneezing, watering of the eyes and nose—a complete catarrh accompanied by a crimson rash, and often attended or followed by inflammation of the mucous membranes of the organs of respiration.

SYMPTOMS.—After a period of incubation, varying from ten to fourteen days, there is a lassitude, shivering, fever and catarrh. The conjunctiva, Schneiderian membrane, mucous membrane of the fauces, larynx, trachea and bronchi, become much affected; swelling of the eyelids; suffused eyes; watery, intolerant to light; sneezing; dry cough; hoarseness; difficulty of breathing; drowsiness, and great heat of the skin; tendency to delirium; frequent hardened and rapid pulse; tongue white-coated. The eruptions come out at the end of the third day; seldom earlier; often later. It consists of small circular dots or spots, like flea bites, which gladly unite into blotches of a dirty-red color, and slightly raised above the skin. The rash first appears upon the forehead and face, and then on the neck and breast, and gradually extends all over the body. It begins to fade away in the same way—first on the forehead, etc. It produces no marked despumation, which is the characteristic of scarlet fever. Diarrhea often sets in on the rash declining. It is usually salutary. The fever does not subside at once on the disappearance of the eruptions; nor does the severity of the attack depend upon the quantity of the rash. The contagion of measles is strong. Pulmonary complications are very apt to follow this disease—laryngitis; cancerum aris; severe otitis; epistaxis; acute tuberculosis, etc.

TREATMENT.—Confine the patient to a warm, dry, airy apartment in bed; enjoin thorough hygenie; have the patient sponged every two or three hours with alkaline warm water or warm vinegar and water, then give the

Tincture of aconite, 10 to 15 drops, in one-third tumblerful of water. Mix.

Tincture of Belladonna, 10 to 15 drops.
Water, one-third tumblerful. Mix.

Dose: Teaspoonful; alternate them every hour.

Occasionally, between times, give warm safron teas, or hot lemonade, and plenty of it. Keep up, if possible, a gentle sweat. Diet—milk, beef tea, butermilk and milk punch (see pages 14 and 17.)

CATARRH.

This is a terrible disease, with which nearly if not quite three-fourths of the human family are afflicted, more or less—from the fact few people ever dream that they have anything but a slight cold or a slight touch of influenza, until all the mucous membranes and air passages are so affected that it has poisoned the blood and assumed a chronic form of one of the most distressing and loathsome diseases, which seems to resist all treatment and is the most difficult to cure. The whole world has been filled with more advertisements of quack nostrums, and perhaps more money spent in this way, for the cure of Catarrh than perhaps any other one disease. Dear reader, let us tell you here that all the money you spend in that way is worse than useless, for you are oftener made far worse than ever benefited, or if you are ever benefited in the least it is only temporary. Catarrh is an inflammation of the mucous membranes of some portions of the air passages, characterized by sneezing, watery discharges from the nostrils, increased secretions from the lachrymal glands, slight head-ache, heavy feeling in the head, chilliness, fever, hoarseness, dry cough, sore throat. Sometimes it assumes to be a drying up of all the secretions, the air passages are all stopped up, and there is a loss of appetite and feeling of lassitude.

Different names are applied to it, as it affects the schneiderian membrane—Catarrhal Cephalgia, when it affects the frontal sinus; Bronchitis, when the stress falls upon the trachea and bronchial tubes. Catarrh, properly speaking, affects the mucous lining of the nose and throat, and is extremely prevalent and intractable. People of a strumous diathesis are most liable to this form of the disease; hence we find the disease of a low chronic type and requiring a specific treatment. If the catarrhal inflammation has been violent in scrofulistic patients, ulceration many times is the result.

The peculiar influences which originate catarrh, affect, primarily, the organic nerves which supply the surface, and through them the system generally. Secretions and the circulation in the parts are specially deranged; the chief modifications of the disease from the constitutional actions are disturbed, the extent of surface involved becomes greater and the grade of iritation proportionately increased.

TREATMENT.—In acute attacks, an emetic of compound powder of lobelia (as described in other parts of this book how to prepare this medicine), followed by a hot air bath and foot bath. Tincture of aconite, given as an arterial sedative, acting freely on the secretions, from ten to fifteen drops to a third of tumblerful of water; dose, teaspoonful every one or two hours, as the case demands. Hot atomized vapors to control the local inflammation. All moist warmth is a powerful restorer in this disease to the arrested circulation and vital action that we possess, and the safest therapeutic agent that we have in this disease, because it is direct. The warm vapors should be allowed to come freely in contact with the inflamed mucous membranes. Various agents are used for inhalations with good success. We feel partial to the sulphate of hydrastis, or Golden Seal, as it is called by the common people; also, the blood-root, or the permanganate potassa. These remedies are all very rapidly absorbed by the mucous membranes; the warm stream softens and relaxes the tissues. There is nothing that acts so promptly as the warm atomizers in catarrh. The atomizing instruments of the various makes can be had at nearly all the drug-stores. Below we will give you a table of remedies to be used and their strength.

The nasal douche is also an indispensable intrument to be used, as it washes out the air passages and keeps them cleansed and prepared to be followed by the medicine for the atomizers. For the douche, various remedies are used in alternation. To a quart of warm water (as warm as can be borne) half a teaspoonful of salt, is a very excellent remedy. Chlorate of potassa, half a drachm to a quart of water, is another. The sulphate of zinc, or diluted carbolic acid, used in various strengths, are very useful. The douche, and how to use it, is too well known to take up the time to describe it here.

The dose in the following table is to be added to an ounce of distilled water for the atomizing instrument. There are many remedies that are used in this way, but we shall give only those which we have had the best success with in the greatest number of different cases. We give these remedies because we do not know the patient to prescribe for him on the spot, leaving you to use such different ones as seem to give the most relief. To use them all alternately will be the best for you:

Sulphate of hydrastin	5 to 10 grains.
Sulphate of baptisin	10 to 20 "
Sulphate of iron	1 to 5 "
Sulphate of sanguinarin	5 to 10 "
Pulv. borax	5 to 20 "
Digitalis	½ to 1 "
Potassa chlorate	5 to 10 "
Potassa bromide	5 to 10 "
Potassa iodide	5 to 10 "
Potassa permanganate	10 to 20 "
Salt	5 to 30 "
Carbolic acid	1 to 7 "
Bichromate of potassa	5 to 10 "

The best of the above is carbolic acid, which stimulates, deoderizes and promotes cicaterization of the abraded surfaces. During this treatment we will give you a prescription of our catarrh snuff; also, a prescription as a blood purifier, that is of the most importance in the cure of this disease:

Fluid extract of the American ivy (ampelopsis quing),

Fluid extract of yellow parilla (menispermum), of each half an ounce.

Fluid extract wild yam root (dioscorea villo), one drachm.

Fluid extract mandrake (podophyllum pelt), half a drachm.

Syrup of stillingia,

Syrup of dandelion, of each equal quantity, sufficient to make a six-ounce mixture.

Mix.

Dose, teaspoonful three times per day.

This is one of the best blood purifiers in catarrhal or scrofulistic conditions that we have ever used, or even in syphilitic diseases. If iodide of potasseum is added two or three drachms, it is still better in syphilitic diseases.

We have a catarrh snuff that we consider the best ever in use. We will give that under the head of "Recipes." See Index.

GONORRHEA.

This is a term applied to inflamation of the mucous membrane of the Urethra, generally beginning at the anterior portion, attended with a contagious mucus, or muco-purulent discharge. The cause is a specific virus of veneral matter coming in contact with the part. Still, leuchorrhea, menstrual discharge, strains or blows may excite a mild type of inflammation, which will pass off in a few days. But true gonorrhea is due to the action of a specific poison depressing the part. It may be a poison of low intensity, or it may be one of great intensity; both forms produce a gonorrhea.

The symptoms of both grades of the poison are identical—no true distinctive mark. Scratch the thigh of the patient and apply a little of the puss; the character of the sore so produced will reveal the type of the virus, the grade of the poison. The period of incubation varies from twenty-four to forty-eight hours after illicit intercourse, sometimes longer, varying with the power of vital resistance of the patient. An itching desire to urinate frequently, heat, fullness and redness of the orifice, slight glary discharge like the white of an egg, which soon becomes muco-purulent, great scalding during micturition, pain in the groin, iritability of the bladder, weight and dragging down of the testicles, are symptoms. However, these symptoms are liable to numerous complications, as cordee, painful erections, balanetis, hemorrhage from the urethra, and retention of urine, abcesses in the groin, prostites etc., etc.

TREATMENT.—This is various. If the patient is seen early, during the first two days, an effort should be made at once to abate the inflammation. If possible, this should be done by injections into the urethra, after each urination, with an injection of sulphate of zinc, grains five, to sulphate of morphia, grains two, to one ounce of water. This will kill the virus at once in two days. Then follow the first by the two following ones:

    Sulphate of hydrastin .... 4 grains.
    Baking soda .... 8 "
    Distilled water .... 3 ounces.

Mix.

Inject after each urination, just a few drops, say half a teaspoonful.

Again:

    Sulphate of hydrastin .... 2 grains.
    Pulverized borax .... 8 "
    Distilled water .... 2 "

Mix.

Inject this alternately with the above. If there are painful erections (cordee), bathe the parts at once in cold water. If it is a simple new case—we mean taken in time—this is all the treatment that is required. But in old cases there will have to be internal treatment, given at the same time the injections are made locally, of the following:

    Compound syrup of stillengia .... 4 ounces.
    Balsam of copaiba .... half "
    Iodide of potassa .... 20 grains.
    Fluid extract of gelsenmum .... half drachm.

Mix.

Dose, teaspoonful three times per day. As soon as the discharges abate take only twice per day. This you can get your druggist to put up for you, and it is good and reliable in such cases. It takes from six days to five or six weeks to cure these cases, according to the condition, constitution, habits and life of the individual.

DIABETES.

This is a real disease which many parents are wholly ignorant of, and therefore many a poor child has been unmercifully whipped to break it from the habit of wetting the bed, which is cruel.

CAUSE.—Diabetes is an affection of the system dependent upon a disordered state of the digestive organs, with a defect of the assimulative functions, which is characterized by a condition of extreme nervous prostration, a morbid appetite for food and drink, and the secretion of a large quantity of glucose, or grape sugar. It is, properly speaking, a saccharine diathesis, for not only is the starch of the food converted into sugar, but, owing to the morbid condition of the liver, or the nerves which supply it, the liver only secretes, *per se*, saccharine elements.

The primary cause of diabetes consists, then, in a morbid condition of the digestive and assimulative organs, which favor the promotion of sugar from the starchy or farinaceous substances introduced into the alimentary canal, and its absorption into the blood and urine. But we cannot enter into the details of the subject in this little book.

TREATMENT.—A regular course of diatetics is of the first importance. A rigid and careful avoidance of all saccharine or starchy articles of food must be observed, and a liberal, nutricious diet must be adopted, consisting of beef, mutton, venison, fowls, game, fish, etc. If the patient can afford it, a sea voyage; if not, a salt-water sponge bath every day, with a brisk and vigorous rubbing down with the hands. Little bits of ice, to allay the intense, craving thirst for drink, should be taken. Buttermilk is good for a drink. [Right here we wish to say, before we forget it, that in all disorders, no matter what, if the stomach will tolerate it, buttermilk is called for as a drink. It will allay thirst as well as water; besides there is a lactic acid in the buttermilk which is good for the stomach; therefore, besides allaying thirst, it is nutricious diet. The author has always prescribed buttermilk in nearly all acute as well as chronic diseases with the most happy and gratifying results.] The body should be well protected with flannels; plenty of exercise in the open air, but never to fatigue. Tonics and alteratives are the medicines in this disease. The best medicine to give is the diluted nitro-muriatic acid, half an ounce to one ounce of glycerine, teaspoonful to a tumbler of water to be used as a drink.

Tincture of nux vomica, four drops; diluted phosphoric acid, eight drops, to half a tumbler of water; dose, teaspoonful every hour for several days, making fresh every day.

Our remedies should all be directed to the head and nervous system, rather than the stomach.

For immediate control of the spasm of the sphincter muscles of the bladder in children who are wetting the bed every night, we will give you several remedies in this disease, as one remedy will not cure every case on account of the peculiar condition of the patient.

You can get at your druggist's Squibb's etherial tincture of ergot; you can give it in from five to ten drop doses, three or four times per day, in a little water. This is very excellent in some cases.

Tincture of iodine, in one-drop doses, three or four times per day.

Tincture of belladonna, from three to five drops doses, on going to bed.

Tincture of gelseminum, from eight to ten drops, on going to bed.

The two last remedies are to be given only on going to bed. One dose per day is all that is required of these two remedies.

ASTHMA.

Asthma is a nervous disease, whose phenomena depend upon a tonic contraction of the circular musclar fibres of the bronchial tubes. Paroxysms induced by direct or reflex mechanism, that is to say, the stimulus to contraction may be central in the medulla oblongata, or it may be in the pulmonary or gastric portion of the pneumogastric, or in some other part of the nervous system. Asthma always has, at the root of it, some central nervous irritation, or some periferal source of it; may be some latent miasma, skin disease, or some organic affection of the chest; while other causes are merely exciting causes, as moist easterly winds. Atmospheric electricity is the inhalation of irritating substances, as the aroma of new mown hay, or malaria, damps, variable climate, incompatibility of the individual to the location; or soil; or country; where he lives, etc.

SYMPTOMS.—A fit of asthma is usually preceded either by headache or sleepiness, or various digestive or other diseases, as lassitude, pain in the head, back or limbs, loss af appetite, dry, hacking cough, depression of spirits. The attack is usually ushered in suddenly during the night, with a sensation of suffocation or constriction about the chest, urgent, distressing dispnœa, aggravated by the slightest movement. Inspirations short and strong, while the expirations are long, labored and loud-wheezing. Great and rapid movements of the nostrils, countenance livid and anxious, indicative of great distress and anxiety, inclined to retain the erect posture, often an intense struggle for breath. On auscultation no respiratory murmer is audible, but vibrating murmer loud and wheezing, or shrill and whistling, pulse small and feeble, eyes staring, and anxious countenance; temperature of surface falls to 82 deg. Fahr.; but after a while the labor and fatigue causes the skin to pour out a most abundant perspiration, and after a period comes relief. At last cough a little with expectoration of little ropy, stringy pellets of mucous and vomits. Paroxysm ceases and the patient falls asleep. During the intervals of attacks the patient usually enjoys good health. It is a frightful sight to any one who never witnessed a person with a spasm of asthma; but it is not a dangerous disease, by any means, for all it is a most distressing one.

There have been many remedies introduced which have, in many cases, afforded temporary relief, such as the common brown paper soaked in a solution of saltpetre, then dried, after which burn it in a tight room, that the patient may inhale the smoke. Also, drying the leaves of the Jamestown weed (stramonium) and smoking them in a pipe or paper. But then they are only temporary relief.

TREATMENT.—When the spasm is on give the patient a teaspoonful of the compound tincture of lobelia every five minutes until relieved, followed with a half drachm dose of bromide potassium. This will seldom fail to relieve the bronchial spasm; but the final cure of asthma lies in the constitutional treatment in the intervals of the attack, by the use of nutritious diets. The alcohol vapor bath three or four times per week, followed by brisk friction with the hands, and regular hygiennic habits; food easily digested; the dyspeptic condition of the stomach must be got rid of, and all the internal organs put in good running order to get rid of this harrassing disease; and the hot air bath will do it if properly administered. The cause must, in all cases, be got rid of, or the patient placed in a location compatible with his idiosyncracies and the closest attention paid to the general health.

Excellent results will be followed by such a prescription as the following:

>   Fluid extract yerba santa (new remedy)... half ounce.
>   Fluid ext. grindelia robusta (new remedy). half ounce.
>   Fluid ext. rosinweed (silphum) .... half ounce.
>   Fluid ext. black cohosh (cimcifuga racem.) 1 drachm.
>   Tincture of lobelia seed........................ half drachm.
>   Bromide potassa................................. half ounce.
>   Hydrocyanic acid, diluted .... 25 drops.
>   Extract of malt .... three and a half ozs.
>   Distilled water sufficient to make a 6-oz. mixture. Mix.

Dose: One teaspoonful one hour after each meal, and one on going to bed, continued for over one week or more.

This prescription, together with the other constitutional treatment that we have given, will effectually cure this disease.

PNEUMONIA.

Pneumonia is an inflammation of the substance of the lungs, and it is predisposed to by intense nervous depressian, debility, or exhaustion. The existing cause is usually the depressing effect of cold, damp, exposure, vicissitudes of heat and cold, or inhalations of irritants, or mechanical violence. The usual mode of attack is depression of the large aerating surface of the lower lobe of the right lung. It may remain there or proceed over to the left lung, and then proceed upward. However, in all conditions, the lungs become engorged from below upwards. Pneumonia may be met with in the following forms: acute, sudden in its character. If the patient has a strong vital force it may resist the local irritation, or it may come down of itself from a slight irritation. In other patients, whose constitutions are feebler, it may involve both pleura and lung, and both be implicated at the same time. Then, again, it may be complicated with typhoid.

But our book is too small to go any farther in detail here. Therefore, we will say that we will have no room to describe Pleurisy, only to say that our treatment would be much the same in both diseases.

TREATMENT.—As soon as the disease is recognized, in either case, the patient should get an alcohol bath and then be put to bed. The temperature of the apartment should be kept between 65 and 70 degs. Active cupping should be resorted to over the consolidated lung, then followed by flaxseed poultices. The action of warmth and moisture over the affected tissues tends directly to increase its vitality, as soon shown by diminished dispnœa, the breath being drawn more easily. Even intercostal movement can be detected. The poultice should be made of linseed meal, because it keeps moist the longest; but it should be fully half an inch thick, spread on flannel sufficiently large to cover the affected part. The poultice should be changed every two hours, as the heat of the body will soon dry it. Then, as the symptoms change for the better you can change the poultice for that of compresses. Take a towel, wring it out dry from a little salt and tepid water, and apply to the chest. Change it often. Lay a dry towel over the wet one. That will prevent the underclothes from getting damp

Remember, you must keep the feet hot and moist by sponging them often with water as hot as can be borne, and give the following prescription as internal treatment:

Fluid extract of pleurisy root (asclepias tuberosa) .... half drachm.
Fluid ext. stone root (collinsonia) .... half drachm.
Fluid ext., sweet bugle weed (lycopus virginicus) .... half drachm.
Water .... three and a half ozs.

Mix.

Dose: Teaspoonful every one or two hours.

If there is much predetermination of blood to the head, give

Tincture of belladonna, 10 to 15 drops.
In half tumbler of water.

Dose: Teaspoonful every hour, alternated with the above medicine, making fresh every day.

This treatment followed out, in a very few days you will be astonished to see how your patient will rally out of this dreaded disease.

Pleurisy can be treated in the same way with success.

How different this treatment from that of the old way, which was always treated by bleeding the patient, followed by mustard drafts, and blistered all over the breast, thus adding more fuel to the already consuming inflammation and heat in the lungs. For their internal treatment was veratum, sweet spirits of nitre, calomel and jalap, carbonate of amonium, the result of which was generally followed by a first-class funeral in the family. The attending physician was always charged with being very attentive during the sickness, and had the credit of handling the patient very skillfully.

GRAVEL.

Gravel may be defined to be the discharge of a gritty powder or sand, or of small calculi deposits passed off with the urine, occasioning pain and irritatian of the kidneys, ureters, bladder and urethra. Gravel is present in the uric, phosphatic and oxalic acid diatheses of the individual. The most common of the three forms is the uric acid—averaging 80 per cent of all the cases. All ages and both sexes are liable to be afflicted with this disease.

THE CAUSE.—Gravel is caused by a false assimilation of the solids and fluids of the body, unhealthy digestive organs, confined to the continued use of soft water or exclusive lime water for both cooking and drinking purposes. Of this, however, the author's opinion is formed from a very extended experience and observation in this disease. In cities where the people cook and drink exclusively cistern water, there is where we have found the most kidney and bladder diseases. We do not believe that anybody should be confined to live exclusively upon either soft or hard water for cooking or drinking purposes, but for health they should use both; but, if we should be compelled to choose one or the other for an exclusive use, we should choose the lime water rather than the usual cistern water; in fact no cistern water is fit to use exclusively for drinking and cooking purposes, unless the cistern has a good filter attached, and there are so few filters that are used that are fit for anything, so far as to filter any of the organic matter out of the water, especially the usual rains that fall in summer, which the people are most generally too apt to catch and save. The falling rains of summer are hardly fit for drinking purposes, as the air is always more or less filled with the carbonicious and malarious poisons that arise from the earth's surface and fill the upper currents of air with its deadly poisons, and as water is one of our best known elements for the absorption of poisons, how can the rain which falls through this atmosphere, help but be filled, more or less, with this poison, which finds its way into our cisterns for drinking purposes, to say nothing of the dirty roofs of our houses, and the filthy gutters and water pipes which are always in every case washed off and out clean from a dashing rain. Now, all of this dirt and poison filth has taken up its quarters in the cistern, to be used by the human body. Now this is all wrong, for nobody can have permanent health living upon this kind of water.

We will give you our plan for a filter, which we have tested to our perfect satisfaction, and know it to be the best filter that we have ever known. It is cheap and durable, and never gets out of order, and we will not charge you anything extra for our patent filter.

When you build your cistern, build it just a little larger than the usual size, especially at the top. Now build you an eight-inch wall right through the center, from picked brick, pretty hard burnt but not too hard, not too soft and shelly, but with nice, square, sharp edges. Lay this eight-inch center wall clear up to the top of your cistern; but it must be laid in mortar made from cement, the same as you use to plaster your cistern with. Strike the joints well; be sure that there are no air holes through between the brick and mortar. Join the center wall to the wall on each side of your cistern. Now, when you plaster it, leave the center wall unplastered, and when your cistern is done let the water pipes in on one side of the wall, and put your pump in on the other side of the wall. Now, as your water runs in the cistern from the rains the water will filter through this eight-inch brick wall, and you will have the purest water that you ever drank, and it will always be pure and free from any kind of organic matter. If you will be choice in the winter and spring to fill your cistern always after a heavy rain, when the roof has had sufficient time to be washed off, you will always have nice, pure, clear water. All cisterns should be cleaned out once per year. This filter will never get out of order, and will last just as long as your cistern will last, and be just about as cheap. This filter can be added to old cisterns, if you will alter the cistern at the top and make it a little bigger, so that any one can put down a ladder, and a man go down to clean it out.

But, bless us! we did not intend to write an article upon cisterns and rain water; but here we have switched entirely off the track and told you how to build cisterns. But for all, it is as good a chapter as there is in the book, so we know the reader will excuse us, while we will try to find our way back to where we started from.

Let's see; we believe we were trying to write an article upon the disease of Gravel, weren't we?

But we will surely have to go back and read over what we said to see where we left off, so that we can pick up the dropped thread, tie a knot and go on.

Gravel, then, as we have said, is caused by an improper assimilation of the fluids of the body, which soon form into sand-like deposits. When the sediments are excessive they are called, chemically speaking, urates; lithates; phosphates, oxalates, according to the diathesis of the patient. When those assimilations are excessive it causes a serious disease, and if there is anything in the bladder like a mucous shred it acts as a nucleus for these sand-like deposits, and it forms what is known as stone in the bladder.

SYMPTOMS.—In Gravel, the patient has a dull, aching pain in the back, preceded by and attended with frequent desire to urinate, followed by sharp, cutting, burning pains in the urethra and neck of the bladder, or in the course of the ureters. These pains extend along down the thigh and into the calves of the legs. The sudden stoppage of the stream of the urine is caused by the stone rolling down into the neck of the bladder, and the patient has a constant desire to be pulling at the end of the penis to relieve the pain, which is always suggestive of the presence of stone in the bladder.

The chemical nature of the gravel should be ascertained, and, when this is done, the chemical opposites in the medicines should be administered, as no treatment will avail if not in chemical opposition. But if the stone has been formed and is of any size, there is no treatment effectual. A surgeon should be consulted, who will remove it by an operation called lithotrity, or another term, lithontripsy.

The solvent treatment consists, of course, of such agents as are chemically opposed to the nature of the calcula deposits. By such a course of medication our success has been the most gratifying.

As soon as the patient is aware, or has the least suspicion that he has the gravel, he should at once see to it that he gets his stomach, as well as all the internal organs, in good running order. A strict nutritious diet should be adhered to. Sponging and bathing is in order and loudly called for. All stimulating drinks should be avoided, and adopt the mucilaginous drinks.

Then the following prescription is a specific to neutralize and get rid of the sand-like deposits. The best remedy that we have ever used for this disease is a tincture made from the inner bark from the root of the sweet apple tree. But the medical properties are only in the root late in the fall and early in the spring, before the sap rises up in the tree, and after it has gone down into the roots. You can make it yourself in the following way, as it seldom ever can be found in the market in the drug stores.

Take of the bark of the root, eight ounces by weight.

Put this into a bottle.

Add alcohol 76° per cent, one pint by measure.

Let it stand from fifteen to twenty days, shaking it occasionally that the strength shall be well drawn out.

Dose of this medicine: One teaspoonful three or four times per day. It can be taken in a little sweetened water.

The next best remedy is the

Fluid extract of hydrangea.

Dose: Fifteen to twenty drops every three hours.

Ten grains of borax dissolved in water, should be drank every day during the treatment.

SPERMATORRHEA.

Under this title it will be necessary to consider Masturbation, or Self-Abuse; Semenal Weakness, Sexual Exhaustion, Sterility, etc.

Masturbation.—Self-Abuse is a name given to a pernicious and destructive habit—a discharge of the seminal fluids by the stimulus of the virile organs with the hand—an act which is revolting to humanity and destructive to every feeling and faculty of vigorous manhood. The great and good in all ages and nations of the world, as well as the highest medical authority, condemn this pernicious, this baneful practice, as fatal to the vitality of the person, entailing on himself a lower type of manhood, and even transmitting to his posterity a structure so degrading that its very constituents are disease, weakness and death. In a very large percentage of nocturnal emissions and enlarged prostate glands, masturbation has been the cause. Nationally speaking, it exercises a disastrous effect, producing imbecility, cerebral diseases of every form, placing the persons lower in the scale of being. But aside from all this general type of degeneration, it creates certain local diseases, such as inflammation of the prostrate glands. This is produced by an unnatural act, being an irritant by the retention of semen in the ejaculatory ducts, producing inflammation. This invariably takes place when the semen is retained—not thoroughly evacuated. Another very common result is the devitalization of the veins of the spermatic cord and testicles, producing a varicose condition of the veins—varicocele and circocele.

Atrophy, or a wasting away of the testicles, is also a very common sequel. This condition may take place at any period. If the practice has been commenced in early life, they often do not attain their natural size, and even lose the power of secreting semen, and thus the manhood is gone forever. But this effect is not on the testicle alone, but upon the whole body, which is bent downward and dwarfed and robbed of its proper proportions—a perfect arrest of any further development. But this subject alone is inexhaustible, and we cannot go any farther into the details only to say that the critical period of life in this disease is about the time of the approach of puberty, which varies from the age of fifteen to eighteen, when the very rapid growth of the generative organs, the increased power and frequent erections cause the act, which is sure to occasion the deepest remorse. It is the attention and deliberate condition of these facts that explain to us how the habitual exercise of the genital organs, either by coition or by masturbation, may so far get control of the will of the individual. It is about this time in life when parents, through an ignorant education combined with a false modesty, have failed to do their duty by not taking the precaution to make confidantes of their boys and girls by talking to them and explaining to their young minds the dangerous period that their lives have about approached and are approaching, by warning them against such a pernicious and loathsome habit. Parents, we warn you to see to it that you do your duty and be ever vigilant and on the watch, before your promising sons are ruined and sent to the mad-house. Do you not know that, according to the statistical evidence which we have, three-fourths of the inmates of our insane asylums are the victims of masturbation? But we cannot follow this subject longer; our book is too small. But we wish we had a voice sufficiently loud that the whole world might hear our warning to you upon this subject.

REMEDY.—First, the habit must at once and forever be abandoned. Without this there is no available remedy. There must be a strict attention paid to the general health, and good, nutritious diet—beef, mutton, fish, eggs, fruit and vegetables. Next, the *mind* must be under complete moral control. You must not think about such things. Get interested in some interesting book, and dwell upon the subject matter read. Seek the society of intelligent, cultured men and women. You must become interested at once in the stern realities and practicabilities of life. Then, and not till then, is there any hope for you.

Through the day you can take the following prescription:

Fluid extract of prickly ash berries (Xanthoxylum), one drachm;
Fluid extract of gelsemium, half drachm;
Fluid extract of hydrastis canad., twenty drops;
Tincture of bayberry bark, half drachm;
Tincture of nux vomica, half drachm;
Glycerine, four ounces.
Mix.

Teaspoonful every three hours during the day time.

If there are nightly dreams, followed by emissions of semen, then the following prescription is for that:

Bromide of potassa, three and one-half drachms;
Hydrate of chloral, three drachms;
Lemon syrup, three and one-half ounces.
Mix.

Dose, teasponful on going to bed only; and remember, don't take any more than this amount unless you find that you do not sleep sound; in that case you can take one and one-half teaspoonfuls at one dose, and take it on going to bed at night only.

SUPPRESSION OF MONTHLY PERIODS (Amenorrhea).

This may occur in three forms: First, where the evacuations have never occurred, or retention of menses; second, where there has never been any secretion; third, suppression.

There are cases where the secretions have been perfect, but the discharge prevented by occlusion of the vagina, or imperfect hymen, etc. Again, the secretions may never have occurred, owing to a congenital deficiency of the ovaries. And there are other cases where the uterus and ovaries are sound, yet no flow from the vagina. The most common variety, however, are when it may cease by degrees, as in consumptive and scrofulous patients; or it may occur as the result of a cold, which induces inflammation of the uterus and ovaries. It may also be induced by excessive venery, or wet feet, ice-water, insufficient clothing, bathing, fear, grief, anxiety, falls, copulation during flow, or pregnancy.

SYMPTOMS.—Weight, pain in the head, loins and uterine regions; hot skin, appoplexy, in some cases various hemorrhages, palpitation of the heart, chilliness, loss of appetite, etc.

TREATMENT.—Give hot alcohol bath, hot foot baths, if the suppression be recent, and apply hot mustard poultices to the breast. Internally, give tansy or wintergreen teas. Keep the patient warm; get her into a sweat; allow but little gentle exercise; give a hot sitz bath, so as to concentrate the blood in the pelvis, putting the feet in a hot bath at the same time. Keep up this treatment for a few days, and all will be well.

DYSMENORRHEA (Painful Menstruation).

Painful menstruation occcurs mostly in single women, and many times it may be pregnancy.

SYMPTOMS.—Restlessness, flushed face, pain in the head, pain in back, pain in the region of the pelvis, sometimes so severe that it will cause fainting; after a while the pain will become more bearing down, accompanied by shreddy mucous discharges, then accompanied by clots of blood. In young and plethoric persons there is but little effect upon the general health, but in very nervous persons the health soon fails, and they not unfrequently run into consumption.

REMEDIES.—When it is thought to be from persistent painful suppression, it is generally pretty certain that it is from an inflammation of the womb. Then the injections are called for, and the local treatment as described on page 48, under the article on "Cause and Cure of Female Weakness."

The use of mild cathartics is necessary to keep the bowels open and free, and the patient should take the following prescription:

Tincture of gelsemium,
Tincture of black cohosh (Cimicifuga racemosa),
Tincture of wild yam (Dioscorea villo), of each half a dram ; *
Glycerine, four ounces.
Mix.

Dose, teaspoonful every three hours.

MENORRHAGIA.

This form of disease is characterized by profuse, prolonged or too freequent menstruation, especially if it is accompanied by head-ache, hot skin, full pulse, weight in the back, hips, loins, and pelvis; the patient becomes bloodless and weak.

CAUSE.—It is occasioned by confinement to hot rooms, abortion, leucorrhea (whites), also excessive venery, long walks, and constipation. Exhaustion follows the least exercise.

TREATMENT.—Locally, injections of a decoction of the plantain leaf, alternated with golden seal (Hydrastis canad.), or a little salt and water; if the hemorrhage is very active, then a strong decoction of tannic acid, or, what is still better, a decoction from the bark of the red oak.

Internally, give the following:

Fluid extract of chamomilla,
Fluid extract of collinsonia,
Fluid extract of ergot,
Fluid extract of sweet bugle weed (lycopus), of each half a drachm ;
Glycerine, four ounces.
Mix.

Dose, teaspoonful every two or three hours, as the case requires, and as improvement is noted prolong the intervals, and when the flow entirely ceases stop the medicine till the next period comes around,

---

* These tinctures can always be had at the Homeopathic pharmacies of a better quality than at any other kind of a drug store; but you must always call for the mother tincture.

while the local treatment should be kept up every day till the diseased condition is healed, after which the patient should have a tonic treatment to build up the lost physical forces, when the following is called for:

Tonic Prescription.—Fluid extract of the tag alder (Alnus rubra),
Fluid extract of wahoo (Euonymus at.),
Fluid extract columbo root (Frasera car), of each half an ounce;
Fluid extract of hydrastis, half a drachm;
Carbonate of iron,
Hypophosphate of lime, of each one drachm;
Table salt, half a drachm;
Good sherry wine (or California angelica wine) and syrup of wild cherry, equal parts, sufficient to make an eight-ounce mixture.
Mix.

Dose, teaspoonful one hour after each meal, and one on going to bed. We consider this one of the best general tonic medicines that ever was given to the world in such cases. You can get your druggist to put it up for you.

CESSATION OF THE MENSES.

This condition usually occurs between the ages of forty and fifty—sometimes later, sometimes earlier. The courses become irregular, staying away two or three months, then commencing with a perfect flood; then again coming scantily, just a show, with sometimes nausea and vomiting, bloating of the abdomen, tenderness of the breasts, etc., are the common symptoms. Pregnancy may sometimes be suspected, for there is frequent uterine pain, dragging-down pains in the back and loins, violent head-ache, sometimes vertigo, a coated tongue and disordered stomach.

TREATMENT.—If the symptoms are light and this change is expected, keep the body in a good condition by strict attention to diet and hygiene, bathing and rubbing the body well three or four times a week. If the pains are in the lower part of the bowels then occasionally wear a pack saturated with equal parts of whisky and water with a little salt added. Internal treatment: Take eight or ten drops of the fluid extract of black cohosh three or four times a day. If the patient is weak and debilitated in general health, then the tonic medicine that we gave you in the other chapter is called for; in fact every indication must be met in the constitutional symptoms.

ST. VITUS' DANCE (CHOREA).

This very singular disease is recognized by a want of control of the muscular nerves over the motor, in the waking state, which gives rise to irregular, tremulous and very ludicrous movements of the voluntary muscles. It occurs, for the most part, in girls of feeble constitutions. About the age of puberty is when it is oftener met with, in girls of irritable, nervous temperament, between the ages of six and fifteen. It is met with very rarely in boys.

CAUSE.—It is from the want of harmony between the gray and white matter of the chord, or it may occur from anemia, dyspepsia, skin eruptions, retarded catamenia, constipation or cold, insufficient food, excessive loss of blood, pregnancy, disease of the bladder or uterus, or mental emotion, etc.

TREATMENT.—This, of all other diseases, has baffled the skill of more physicians than any other, and yet it is more easy and simple for us to cure than any other disease, because we have, in nearly all cases, found the symptoms of nearly a complete congestion of the entire capillary system. Hence, we have directed our treatment almost entirely to the surface of the body; first sponging the body with tepid water, followed by anointing the body with goose grease or a liniment lotion, which we intend to give under the head of Receipts and Prescriptions. Look for it. After several days of this treatment give alcohol sweat baths two or three times per week, with good rubbing and friction with the hand, of the entire body, with occasional anointing, as human magnetism from a gentle, loving hand, is the all important potent remedy in this disease. The bowels must be kept open, and strict attention paid to the diet of good, nutritious food, is all that is necessary in the treatment of this disease.

CATALEPSY.

This is a periodical disease, in which the attack is marked by unconsciousness and fixed rigidity of all or many of the voluntary muscles, so that patients remain in the position they had taken when the attack began. The attack generally lasts but a few minutes. This disease attacks mostly the female sex. Exceptional cases are on record where the attack has lasted several days. At the end of the attack the patient awakens as from a deep sleep, and will take up the sentence in which he was interrupted by the attack, no matter how long it may have lasted. This disease is of very rare occurrence.

TREATMENT.—This must be alterative; tonic and hygienic, and be governed by the general principles which govern us in the forms of diseases with which it is associated. Usually we have had the most satisfactory results from the alternate use of hot and cold water poured on the back of the neck from a height. Internally give phosphorus, quinine and iron in alternation. Doses of three drops of the tincture of the calabar bean every two hours.

EPILEPSY.

This is a chronic disease, and consists of periodical convulsions, unconsciousness and loss of feeling during the attack. This dreadful disease is the most prevalent of all diseases, as statistics prove that one person out of every thousand is a subject of epilepsy.

CAUSES.—Heriditary transmission, intemperance, venereal excesses, self-abuse, blows on the head, fright, and the effects of heat during hot weather.

SYMPTOMS.—Warning of the attack occurs, in a minority of cases, by headaches, dizziness, terror, spectral illusions, or the epileptic aura. This is a sensation like a current of air, and begins either in a hand or foot, or in the spine, proceeding towards the brain. In the largest majority of cases the attack commences with a violent scream, the patient falls down unconscious and convulsions occur. Foaming at the mouth, grinding of the teeth and biting of the teeth, are common; the face becomes bluish-purple, and there are erratic, involuntary muscular movements. Breathing is generally very labored. The duration of the fits is from five to ten minutes. The interval between the attacks may be from several months to a few hours. We have had patients who had several attacks daily.

TREATMENT.—During the intervals and to cure, we should improve the general health with good diet, exercise in the open air, by daily bathing, occasionally vapor bath, etc.; and, above all things, we should endeavor to suspend the explosion of the nervous system with large doses of bromide of potassium in doses from ten grains to a drachm two or three times daily, and continue till we effect cure by other means. We have had great success in curing many cases of this kind with the bromide of calcium, and the bromide of ammonium, and the bromide of lithium, in from one grain doses up to twenty grains, three or four times per day. Sometimes we use one and sometimes the other. The bromide of calcium is an excellent remedy in the convulsions of little children during dentition and diarrhea or vomiting. It takes the place of all other sedatives in doses from one to twenty grains. One grain for every year up to twenty years, is the standard dose.

But in this disease we have had some happy results from the following prescription:

Camphor water, four ounces.
Bromide of potassium, one ounce.
Bromide of ammonia, one-half ounce.
Potass. bicarbonate, two drachms.
Tincture of calabar bean, one-half ounce.
Tincture of belladonna, thirty drops.
Mix.

Dose: A teaspoonful every three hours.

If the disease is clearly connected with other causes, which only give rise to reflex irritation, or of syphilitic, or mercurial, or any other morbid condition of the blood, our treatment is always attended with decided success. But if the disease depends upon exostosis on the interior of the skull, or upon some organic disease, we can do but little—only to mitigate its severity.

PARALYSIS.

This disease consists of a partial or total loss of voluntary motion or sensation; in some cases both are destroyed. It usually occurs without coma, or loss of consciousness or derangement of the intellectual powers, unless it be, perhaps, merely a derangement of memory. It may be called general when it affects the whole body, and sometimes it is followed by apoplexy. It appears generally suddenly, without any warning by previous symptoms. Most generally only one side of the body is attacked, and the patient loses the power of motion and sensation; and then, again, it is only one arm or one leg that is attacked, and then it may extend to other parts of the body.

CAUSE.—Brain affection, inflammation or effusion, abscess, softening, or blood poisoning of some kind, by opium or tobacco, diseases of the kidneys, chorea, also diseases of the spinal chord, excessive sexual appetite, masturbation, etc.

TREATMENT.—If the patient is young and vigorous, a most active course of treatment should be pursued, so as to diminish the pressure on the brain. Mustard applied from the extremities to the knees, with strict attention paid to diet and hygiene, bathing and frictionising the body with the hands; in fact this is a stubborn disease to deal with, and human magnetism is the most potent remedy that we know of in this disease. It will yield to the magnetic treatment from the loving hand of a friend when it will yield to no other treatment. You must have confidence as well as patience in this disease, and treatment for it is slow to yield. The affected parts should be manipulated well with the hand, and lastly passes made all the way down from the top of the head down the spine to the feet, for half an hour, after the other parts have been vigorously treated by rubbing well.

Electricity is also good in this disease, but it must be applied by one who thoroughly understands the application of it.

The following prescription we have always found the best that we have ever used for this disease:

Oil of olive, one ounce.
Oil of cinnamon,
Oil of cloves, of each one drachm.
Muriate of ammonia, two and a half drachms.
Aqua opium,
Alcohol, of each two ounces.
Water, sufficient to make a four-ounce mixture.
Mix well.

Now apply this lotion to the affected parts twice a day with the hand, and rub it in well.

DYSPEPSIA.

This disease occurs with different diseases of the stomach in part, and also partly as a symptom in conditions, the causes of which have never been satisfactorily explained.

SYMPTOMS.—The manifestations are very similar, in many cases, to catarrh of the stomach—pressure and a sensation of fulness in the region of the stomach, bloating, appetite is diminished, sometimes there is aversion to all kinds of food, and great desire for pickles and highly seasoned dishes. Digestion is much slower than usual. Food is often vomited several hours after a meal, not digested at all or penetrated with acidity or gases, producing flatulence, which finds relief by belching. The bowels are generally costive. Dyspepsia is not a dangerous, but generally a very obstinate disease.

CAUSES.—Overfilling the stomach with large quantities of food, impairing digestion. Too large quantities of cold or warm water. All articles of food which lessen digestion, such as coffee, tea and spirituous beverages, and those also which are easily transposed into acids or vinegar, or butter, or which have already changed in part before eating, rich or sour milk, sour beer, sour wine, old cheese and spoilt meat.

Dyspepsia may also be formed in all febrile diseases, with scrofula, diabetes, etc., and may also originate after diseases of the nerves and mind.

TREATMENT.—Diet is of the greatest importance in the treatment of dyspepsia. Only very easily digestible articles of food are to be allowed. To these belong flour and milk soups, very thin beef tea, buttermilk, raw or very soft boiled eggs, game, pigeons, white meats, soft smoked ham, wheat bread; but, on the contrary, the following are hard to digest and to be avoided: All hulled vegetables, as beans, peas, etc., rye bread, cake, fat meats, fat soups, hard smoked ham, etc. The patient is only allowed to take small quantities at a time, never fill his stomach full, and never eat until fully satisfied. Patients are only allowed to eat again when we can judge that the food previously taken is perfectly digested and has passed through the stomach. With healthy grown people this takes place in from four to six hours, but with dyspeptics a much longer time is needed. The dyspeptic should eat only very plain food, and avoid many varieties of food at one meal. He also should not eat late evenings, nor go to bed with a full stomach. Much drinking of cold water is especially to be avoided. An important point of the treatment lies in a perfect regularity of habits, as eating, sleeping, etc.

Then the following prescription is in order, and will do you good service:

Fluid extract of columbo root,
Fluid extract of tag-alder, of each one-half ounce.
Fluid extract of hydrastis, one-half drachm.
Diluted phosphoric acid, three drachms.
Tincture of nux vomica, one-half drachm.
Syrup of wild cherry,
Syrup of lemon, of each sufficient to make a six-ounce mixture.
Mix.

Dose: Teaspoonful after each meal, and one on going to bed.

DROPSY.

This is a disease too deep to go into the details of its history and causes for the space of our little book, farther than to say that it may become partial or general in its manifestations. The main cause is from the large venous trunk being compressed, or obliterated, so that the blood can no longer circulate through it, while the collateral vessels can not be relieved; hence dropsical effusion is the result, and the effusion is in proportion to the size and importance of the vein obliterated or compressed. If, for instance, in the vena cava, or large vein in the abdomen, compression or any other obstacle should prevent the return of the blood, then the two lower intestines, as well as the scrotum, would become filled with water, or serum, and collections may perhaps also take place in the abdomen. Then again, if this obstruction takes place at the very center of circulation, namely, the heart, in this case the return of blood everywhere would become embarrassed; then the dropsical effusion would become general. A cold will often produce dropsy, as will also eruptive skin diseases, such as scarlet fever, or rheumatism, or it may result from degeneration of the kidneys, or from glandular enlargement of the liver, etc., etc. Albumen is always present in the urine in this disease. This can be discovered by boiling the urine in a small tube, the albumen becoming like the white of an egg boiled.

SYMPTOMS.—In the first stages, weakness and dyspepsia, and the blood loses its red particles very rapidly, but there is little to call attention to the kidneys. Then, in the second stages, the symptoms are a pallid, pasty complexion, and often a dry, hard skin; drowsiness, weakness, indigestion and frequent nausea, often retching the first thing in the morning, and often palpitation of the heart. A most characteristic symptom is that the patient is awakened several times during the night with a desire to make water.

TREATMENT.—This is one of those harrassing complaints which physicians who are in family practice seldom have the patience to investigate and manage with sufficient care. The condition of the stomach, bowels and skin should have special attention. Free action of the skin should be had, as in this way the kidneys are relieved, and thus the blood is purified. Stimulating diuretics should not be used, but, to get up a free diuresis, resort at once to the hot-air bath two or three times a week, followed by oiling the body well with goose grease or olive oil, rubbing it in well with the hands. A counter irritation should be made over the region of the kidneys.

It is our confident belief that this grave disease can be cured in nearly every instance if not too far advanced. We know it from the success that has always attended our treatment. We will cheerfully and gladly attend any of our readers in the place where we are at work selling our book, who may have this disease. We will now give you a prescription for this disease, to be given during the other treatment which we have just given you. It has always given us the most happy results:

    Fluid extract of unicorn root (Helonin),
    Fluid extract of Indian hemp (Apocynum cannabinum), of each one-half ounce;
    Glycerine sufficient to make a four-ounce mixture.
    Mix.

Dose, teaspoonful every two or three hours, as the case will demand. If the stomach is weak and will not tolerate the medicine without nausea, then take less of it at a dose and oftener.

INTERMITTENT FEVER.

This disease is commonly called Fever and Ague, or Chills and Fever, as the name implies. It is too well known by the common people to need any description by us. It is distinguished by the physicians under the following names: Quotidian, if the fit of chills and fever return every day; Tertian, if the fit comes on every third day; Quartan, if it comes on every fourth day. The length of the intervals determines the variety of Ague, and when those varieties duplicate, then they are called Double Quotidian, etc., etc.

This disease should not be allowed to run long, but should have prompt and efficient treatment at once, as it is liable to run into a chronic form and the liver and spleen and kidneys become seriously affected, and sometimes dropsy is the result. We have no doubt that this disease in the past has caused more harrassing trouble to the old-school physicians to get control of and cure, than perhaps all other fevers combined; yet it is the most simple and easy disease for us to cure, and we will guarantee to cure it every time without the use of quinine, either. So here is the prescription and treatment:

    Fluid extract of Grindelia squarrosa,
    Fluid extract of Eucalyptus globulus, of each one ounce;
    Fluid extract of Baptisia tinctora, one drachm;
    Fluid extract of Podophyllum peltatum,
    Tincture of nux vomica, of each half drachm;
    Glycerine sufficient to make a six-ounce mixture.
    Mix.

Dose, teaspoonful every three hours, for a day or so then three times per day until it is all taken.

During this time you must take three or four alcohol sweats (as described on page 29, in which we describe our bath-box), followed each time by a good, brisk rubbing. This treatment alone will cure this disease every time, *sure*.

Dr. Jones' Home Turkish Bath.

As partially described on page 28, the following dimensions will show how each family can make a Turkish Bath of their own at a trifling expense, from lumber that is plowed and grooved, five-eighths of an inch in thickness:

Four feet high, 3 feet 6 inches long, 2 feet 3 inches wide—all inside measurement; 18 inches high in front up to the door; 8 inches from the back of the bath to the edge of the hole which receives the neck; hole for the neck, 5 inches in diameter; from the edge of the hole in front of that to the door, 6 inches—this will give you the slant of the door. There must be a slot cut in front of the hole for the neck, 5 inches wide, so that when the bather seats himself on the seat in the bath-box his neck can go back through this slot to the hole prepared for the neck; this slot must be fitted in, after the bather is in position, with a block with tongue and groove, so that when it is slipped to its place it will fit the neck nicely. Then you can shut the door, and all is in readiness to proceed with your bath.

The water tank should be as high up and as far away from the bath box as convenient, so as to get all the fall or force from the water through the spray, which should strike the bather with as much force as he can bear. However, all can see at a glance the bath box, bather, water tank, and faucet with hose attached, without any further description.

94 PEARLS OF WISDOM,

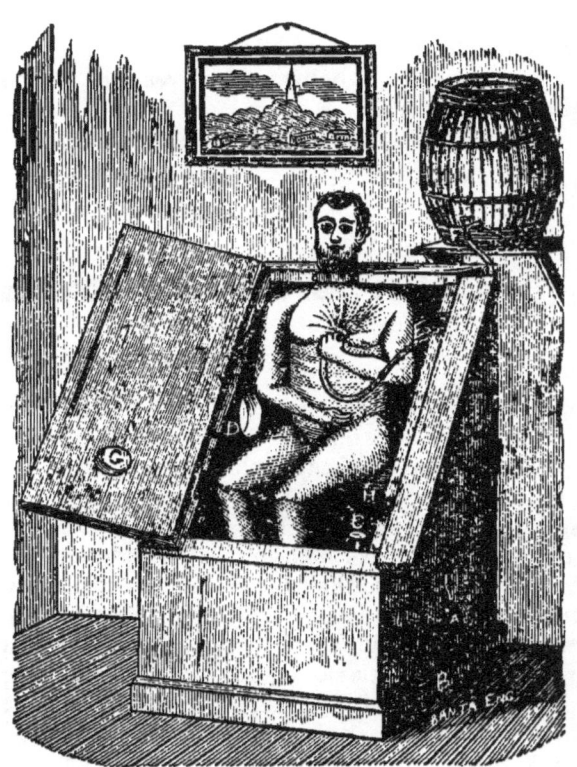

H represents the seat, a stool which is made to raise or lower at will. D, small slide door, in front of which, on the outside of the bath box, is a small shelf attached to hold soap, sponge, brush, and such other things as the bather will need, and to which, by pushing back the slide door, he can help himself at will when he takes a bath without an attendant. G, slide door in the main door, through which to pour additional hot water in the foot bath when required. A, slide door to admit the alcohol lamp under the patient when you want to take an alcoholic sweat, or Turkish bath, as it is called. E, India rubber hose, which is attached to the water tank, on the other end of which is attached a very finely punctured spray nozzle, which can be procured at the plumber's or gas-fitter's. C, stop-cock to let the wastewater run away into the waste-pipe or drain. B, iron pan, large enough to set the bath-box inside of it, to catch the water in case you should desire to give an invalid a bath in a bed chamber or on a parlor carpet.

This is a portable bath, and costs but little to build. Any one can see at a glance the practicability of such a bath arrangement. For cleansing purposes it is unequaled, as the bather can rinse himself off first with the spray, then soap or lather himself thoroughly. By having the top of the bath-box on hinges to turn back, he can stand up and spray himself off as much or as long as he chooses; or he can sit down on a low stool, shut himself all up in the bath, and spray himself off, the water running on him in imitation of a hard shower of rain, and running off in the waste-pipe all the while. In this way you get more benefit from the water than to lie down in it; therefore it is more scientific.

Besides all these advantages, we have a combination bath-tub all in one. We can give a better Turkish bath in this box at your own home than you can get in any large city in the world, for, inasmuch as there are many who cannot stand the hot air on their heads, you can take the hot air sweat with the head outside of the box; or, you can sit on a low stool, shut the bath-box all up, and in this way you have the real Turkish bath, only better in every way. Then you can give the vapor bath, the electrical bath, the sulphur fume bath, and the medicated vapor bath, all in this one box, each of which can be followed by the spray bath. The water can be warmed by the stove, and be prepared to suit the taste previous to taking the bath.

Recipes, Etc.

CONSTIPATION OF THE BOWELS.

INFALLIBLE PRESCRIPTION.

Fluid extract of cascara sagrada, one ounce.
Fluid extract of grindelia squarrosa,
Fluid extract of berberis aquifolium, of each one-half ounce.
Fluid extract of podophylum peltatum,
Tincture of nux vomica, of each one-half drachm.
Citric acid, one-half drachm.
Glycerine, two and one-half ounces.
Mix.

Dose: Teaspoonful after each meal and on going to bed.

This medicine acts slow at first, but when once its action takes place, then less quantity of the medicine is required—taken twice per day, or once per day, or it can be taken once every other day, but the medicine must be taken regular enough to have the bowels move under its influence, till the medicine is all taken up. This will cure those persistent cases of constipation effectually as no other prescription ever did. It is invaluable. It is worth more than the price of a dozen books like this. The fluid extract of cascara sagrada of Park, Davis & Co.'s manufacture, we have always found the best preparation. The cascara is good for dyspepsia; taken in small doses we consider this one of the most valuable remedies ever given to medical science.

FOR COMMON BILIOUS CONDITION.

Tincture of gelsemium,
Tincture of nux vomica, of each one drachm.
Citric acid, one-half drachm.
Sulphate of quinine, thirty grains.
Glycerine, two and one-half ounces.
Mix.
Dose: Teaspoonful in a little water after each meal.

CHOLERA INFANTUM.

Tincture of nux vomica,
Tincture of ipecac,
Tincture of baptisia, of each ten drops.
Tincture of aconite root, five drops.
Lactopeptine, one-half drachm.
Glycerine,
Aqua camphora, of each two ounces.
Mix.

Dose to a child eighteen months or two years old: Give teaspoonful every half hour till relieved, then prolong the intervals.

If the child is very restless and does not sleep well, you may give the following:

Bromide of potassium, two drachms.
Fluid extract of gelsemium, twenty drops.
Glycerine, two ounces.
Mix.

Dose: Half a teaspoonful every half or one hour till the child gets quiet or goes to sleep, then stop this medicine till the child gets restless again.

Remember, all the prescriptions under this head you can get your druggist to put up for you. These medicines should be marked what they are for, and put away carefully and kept through the summer, to be used as occasion requires.

CATARRH OF THE BLADDER.

The common skunk bush (ustilago maydis or rhus aromatica.)
Fluid extract, of Park, Davis & Co.'s manufacture.
Teaspoonful at a dose, in a little sweetened water, three or four times a day; as the symptoms improve prolong the intervals.

For diabetes (insipidus)—children wetting the bed—take
Rhus aromatica, one ounce.
Glycerine, two ounces.
Water, one ounce.
Mix.
Dose: Teaspoonful every three or four hours, as the case may demand.

This is a new remedy, introduced to the profession by Dr. McClanahan. He says that for all of those bladder troubles this remedy alone surpasses all others. It has been well endorsed by many other eminent physicians as accomplishing all that Dr. McClanahan claims for it. We have had no case nor occasion to try it yet.

MALARIAL AFFECTIONS.

Tincture of iodine, ten drops in a third of a tumbler of sweetened water at one dose, three times per day, cures it better and quicker than quinine. For children, give proportionate doses.

RHEUMATISM.

Iodide potassium, one-half ounce.
Solid extract conium, two drachms.
Syrup aralia, compound of American Dispensatory, six ounces.
Mix.

Dose: Teaspoonful three times per day.

Dr. Pitzer says this will never fail to cure any kind of muscular rheumatism.

HOW TO PREVENT A FELON.

It is unnecessary for any one to have a felon if the white of an egg and half a teaspoonful of salt is applied in time. It will scatter it at once. We have tried it many times with success. But if it is not done in time it will do no good.

But the following prescription will draw it to the surface very quickly:

Take equal parts of brown soap and unslaked lime, equal parts of whisky and common kerosene, until a salve is made, and bind it on the felon. In twenty-four hours it will draw the matter to the surface, when it can be removed.

BONE FELONS, CARBUNCLES AND BOILS.

To allay the pain in these distressing comforters use the following prescription:

Tincture of aconite root,
Tincture of arnica,
Tincture of cantharides,
Tincture of veratrum, of each two drachms.
Tincture of iodine, three drachms.
Mix.

Saturate a cotton cloth and apply to the parts, and keep it wet with the mixture till the pain ceases, and give twenty-drop doses of the arnica every hour.

POISON OAK OR IVY.

Cosmoline, one ounce.
Bromine, one-half drachm.
Mix.

Apply to the affected parts two or three times a day. Wash off the medicine twice a day with a little castile soap and soda water, and on going to bed apply the medicine thoroughly. Warm the cosmoline so that the bromine will mix well, then keep the bottle well corked and setting bottom side up, as the bromine will escape upwards.

CHAPPED HANDS, FACE OR LIPS.

Cosmoline is the most excellent of anything that we have ever used. Apply it several times a day.

CONVULSIONS IN LITTLE CHILDREN.

Bromide of sodium, forty grains.
Simple syrup, one-half ounce.
Camphor water, one-half ounce.
Mix.
Dose: Teaspoonful every two or three hours.
For a child three years old, three grains of bromide of sodium in a little simple syrup, three times a day.

SUMMER DIARRHEA IN LITTLE CHILDREN.

From eighteen months to five years old, give them
Sugar of milk, one-half ounce.
Lactopeptine, fifteen grains.
Hydrochloric acid,
Lactic acid, of each one-half drachm.
Tincture of prickly ash berries (Xanthoxylum), one drachm.
Syrup of lemon,
Water, of each one ounce.
Mix.
Dose: Teaspoonful every hour, or half a teaspoonful every half hour is better, and as the symptoms improve prolong the intervals.

FOR RICKETY CHILDREN.

For little children whose muscles are flabby, whose bones are weak and who seem not to grow strong, give them
Hypophosphite of lime,
Hypophosphite of potassium, of each one drachm.

Hydrochloric acid,
Fluid extract of yellow root (Hydrastis) of each one-half drachm.
Lactopeptine, one-half drachm.
Syrup of rhubarb, one-half ounce.
Syrup of lemon, three ounces.
Mix.

Dose: Teaspoonful three times a day. Bathe your child in soda water; alternate it with a little salt and water.

RHEUMATIC GOUT.

Tincture of blue flag (iris versicolor) three drachms.
Tincture of prickly ash, (Xanthoxylum) one drachm.
Glycerine, four ounces.
Mix.

Dose: Teaspoonful three times a day. Sponging and bathing the body are always called for in this disease.

PROFUSE MENSTRUATION.

Fluid extract of ergot,
Fluid extract of hammamelis, of each one drachm.
Fluid extract of Indian hemp (cannabis Indica) two and one-half drachms.
Fluid extract of black cohosh (Macroty's) one drachm.
Glycerine, three ounces.
Mix.

Dose: Teaspoonful every one or two hours as the case requires, or it can be taken every half hour in urgent cases. As the symptoms improve prolong the intervals.

PAINFUL MENSTRUATION.

Fluid extract wild yam (dioscorea vil.) one and a half drachms.
Fluid extract of gelseminum, one drachm.
Tincture of aconite root, 10 drops.
Glycerine,
Water, of each two ounces.
Mix.

Dose: Teaspoonful every hour till relieved, then prolong the intervals.

EXCESS OF VOMITING.

Tincture of nux vomica, from two to five drops.
Tincture of ipecac, from ten to fifteen drops.
Water, four ounces.
Mix.
Dose: Teaspoonful every half hour.
Also, a weak decoction of peach tree leaves, or apple tree leaves, taken alternately with the above will do the work.

NIPPLE WASH. (Dr. Attler's Celebrated).

Powdered borax, one drachm.
Gum Arabic, two drachms.
Tincture of myrrh, three drachms.
Distilled water, four ounces.
Mix.
Apply to the sore nipples two or three times a day.

NURSING SORE MOUTH.

Pure rain water, one-half gallon.
Pulverized yellow root (Hydrastis), one ounce.
Burnt alum, one ounce.
Table salt, one ounce.

While you are burning the alum, and while it is bubbling, sprinkle the salt over the alum. Mix all together with the juice of two lemons and let stand in the sun three or four days, shaking occasionally. Apply to the gums and ulcers with a cotton rag two or three times a day. If it is too strong for the sore parts, weaken with a little sugar and water.

Dr. J. Bobb says this never fails to cure these troubles.

INTERNAL MEDICINE FOR SAME.

Neutralizing cordial, of American Dispensatory, four ounces.
Fluid extract of stone root (collinsonia),
Fluid extract of hydrastis canadensis, of each two drachms.
Fluid extract of black cohosh, (Macroty's).

Fluid extract of white snake root, (eupatorium aromaticum), of each one-half ounce.

Mix.

Dose: Teaspoonful three or four times per day. For the child, weaken it accordingly.

TONIC FOR DISEASE OF THE KIDNEY.

Balsam of Fir, three ounces.
Balm of Gilead buds, fresh ones, two ounces.
Linn bark, one ounce.

Steep the buds and bark slowly in sufficient water to get the strength out of the medicine, in a covered vessel. Then strain and add sufficient sugar to make a pint of the mass. Now cut the balsam with a pint of good Holland gin, by shaking thoroughly. Then add the syrup of the buds and bark, and shake well.

Dose: Teaspoonful three or four times a day.

This is one of the most valuable tonics for diseases of the kidney, with constant pain in the back, we have ever used. It is invaluable.

INACTION OF THE KIDNEYS.

Fluid extract of queen of the meadow, (eupatorium purpureum) one-half ounce.
Fluid extract of pleurisy root (aclepias tub.) one drachm.
Fluid extract of blood root (sanguinaria cana) twenty drops.
Nitrate of potass., two and a half drachms.
Syrup of lemon,
Syrup of ginger, of each two ounces.
Mix.

Dose: Teaspoonful every three hours.

This prescription is very excellent following rheumatism or malarial fevers to set free the poison in the blood and carry it out of the system through the kidneys.

DIPHTHERIA.

Dialyzed iron, two drachms;
Chlorate of potassa, one drachm;
Tincture of iodine, five drops;
Distilled water, half ounce;
Glycerine, one and one-half ounces.
Mix.

Dose, to a child five years old, half a teaspoonful in a little sweetened water, every one or two hours, as the case demands.

FOR EXTERNAL APPLICATION.

Fluid extract of belladonna, two ounces;
Hydrate of chloral, half ounce;
Glycerine, half ounce.

Dissolve the chloral in two ounces of water; then mix all together. Now apply this on the outside of the throat with a cotton cloth, and a flannel cloth over that.

ERYSIPELAS.

Dialyzed iron, half ounce;
Tincture of iodine, ten drops;
Sulphate of quinine, twenty grains;
Glycerine, one and one-half ounces.
Mix.

Dose, half a teaspoonful in a little water every three hours.

In this disease, remember, the bowels must be kept open by cathartics, or injections of a little salt and water.

For external treatment in erysipelas, use the following prescription:
Sulphate of soda, two drachms;
Tincture of wild yam (Dioscorea vill.),
Tincture of veratrum vir.,
Tincture of lobelia seed, of each two drachms;
Distilled water, four ounces.
Mix.

Wet a cotton cloth in this mixture and lay it on the affected parts and keep it moist with the medicine. If the disease is on the face, care should be taken not to get any of the medicine in the eyes.

RHEUMATISM.

Iodide of potassa, five drachms;
Solid extract of conium, two drachms;
Syrup of aralia (the compound of the American Dispensatory), six ounces.
Mix.

Dose, teaspoonful three or four times per day.

Dr. Pitzer says this will cure rheumatism when all other remedies fail. We have never tried it.

DRESSINGS FOR BURNS AND ULCERS.

Carbolic acid, half drachm;
Cosmoline, three ounces;
Balsam of Fir, two ounces;
Water, one ounce.

Warm the cosmoline first; then mix the balance and stir till cold. Apply this to the burn or ulcers as a dressing.

EAR-ACHE.

Glycerine of tannin, half ounce;
Tincture of laudanum, twenty drops;
Sulphate of hydrastin, two grains;
Sulphuric ether, one drachm.
Mix.

Drop three or four drops of this medicine in the ear, from off the end of a little stick is the best. We have never known this to fail in a single instance to cure this distressing disease in children in a very few minutes.

FOR THE ITCH.

Oil of bergamot, half ounce;
Glycerine, one and one-half ounces.
Mix.

Apply in the evening and wash off in the morning with a little soda-water and soap. Pleasant and effectual. (Dr. Yaunkin.)

LOST APPETITE.

Tincture of Apocynum canabinum (Indian hemp), half drachm;
Tincture of Hydrastis canad., one drachm;
Elixir of vitriol, three drachms;
Simple syrup, four ounces.
Mix.

Dose, teaspoonful after each meal.

Magnetic Liniment, for Rheumatism, Sprains, or Stiff Joints.

Oil of lavender,
Oil of sassafras,
Oil of cedar,
Oil of organum,
Oil of spearmint,
Aqua ammonia, fff, of each two ounces.

The whites of three eggs, well mixed and cut with half a pint of alcohol. Dilute a little part of it with water, and pour on the eggs, little at a time, and shake hard; then pour on a little more and shake, and so on, as the alcohol will cook the eggs if it is poured on full strength and all at once. Then, after the eggs are well amalgamated, add all of the balance of the ingredients at once; then add half an ounce of tincture of camphor. Shake well every time you use it, as the mixture separates on standing. This is the most valuable liniment ever given to the world for this purpose. It must be kept well corked, as the medicine will evaporate. You must apply it with the hand, and rub it in well. Don't be in a hurry; take plenty of time in applying it, as the medicine is slow in penetrating the muscles and membranes. The author has made many remarkable cures with this liniment, after all hopes of the patient had fled.

Magnetic Lotion, or Liniment, for the Human Body.

Oil of amber,
Oil of lavender,
Oil of organium,
Oil of sassafras,
Oil of spearmint, of each, half ounce;
Oil of olives, one ounce;
Spirits of turpentine, half ounce;
Aqua amonia, half ounce;
Tincture of opium, one ounce;
Alcohol, not quite one pint.
Mix.

This lotion is most excellent for bathing the chest or the entire body of persons of weak lungs, or anybody that is weak from loss of vitality; or it is splendid for all kinds of sore throat, to bathe the throat well with it, then saturate a flannel with the medicine and pin it around the throat. Some of our patients have pronounced this remedy splendid for rheumatism, or sprains, and weak back.

DR. JONES' RESTORATIVE COMPOUND.

FOR INTERNAL OR EXTERNAL USE.

Good for Cholera Morbus, Nervous Headache, and all kinds of relaxed conditions of the Bowels:

Oil of organium,
Oil of sassafras, of each, one ounce;
Pure sweet spirits of nitre, three ounces;
Saturated tincture of camphor, one ounce;
Essence of peppermint, two drachms;
Fluid extract of capsicum, one drachm;
Chloroform, three ounces;
Aqua amonia, fff, two ounces;
Ninety-eight per cent alcohol, half a pint.
Mix, and keep well corked.

For sprains bruises, rheumatism, or weak back, bathe the parts well with the medicine, applied with the hands.

To treat a case of cholera, the medicine takes the place of a mustard draft, by wetting the hand (or a piece of silk oil-cloth is still better) and laying it on the stomach, wrists and bottoms of the feet, taking care to hold the hand still, excluding all the air from the body and hand where it is applied, and give a half teaspoonful internally every ten or fifteen minutes, as directed for internal use below. Frictionize the body all over well with the medicine, by rubbing with the hands lively till the body smarts or feels hot; then cover the patient all up in a dry, hot blanket.

For nervous sich head-ache, bathe the temples, back of the ears and neck, and a little on top of the head. Smell the medicine occasionally, and take half a teaspoonful every ten or fifteen minutes, as per directions for internal use.

FOR INTERNAL USE.

The medicine must be prepared as follows:

To one teaspoonful of the medicine add two of water; mix in a tumbler, stir up well, and must be mixed as it is used, as it loses its qualities by exposure to the air. Keep the bottle well corked.

For Chronic Diarrhœa—Dose, one teaspoonful to one and a half, as the case requires, from every half hour to four and six hours.

For children, the medicine must be weakened by adding more water and a little sugar, according to the age of the child, and as your judgment dictates.

N. B.—Remember, this medicine must never be taken *internally full strength*, as it will burn your stomach.

This medicine is invaluable, and should be kept on hand in every family. The author has saved the life of many a person with this medicine, who would have died had we not had it on hand. It is the most valuable of all medicines in such cases as described above. The medicine is always in great demand wherever the author is known.

CATARRH SNUFF.

Powdered bayberry root, one and one-half drachms;
Powdered galangal root, one and one-half drachms;
Powdered valerian, thirty-six grains;
Powdered blood root, sixteen grains;
Powdered camphor gum, fifteen grains;
Powdered burnt alum, thirty-six grains.
Mix, and triturate all together well.

Snuff a little of this up the nostrils three or four times per day. It is the best snuff that we have ever used for catarrh, followed by the nasal douche once per day.

Powders for Cramps in the Stomach or Bowels, or Diaphoretic Powder.

Powdered opium, ten grains;
Powdered ipecac, twenty-five grains;
Powdered camphor, forty grains;
Powdered saltpetre, two and one-half drachms.
Mix, and triturate well all together.

From three to five grains to a dose, repeated, if necessary, every three or four hours. Dr. Scudder says this is most excellent in all such cases.

DYSENTERY—BLOODY FLUX.

Fluid extract of chamomile, one drachm;
Fluid extract of epilobium ("wake up willow" herb), one drachm;
Fluid extract of crane's-bill (geranium), half drachm;
Fluid extract of saffron (Crocus satava), one drachm;
Fluid extract of Seneca snake root (Polygala Seneca), two drachms;
Camphor gum, five grains;
Pulverized opium, twenty grains;
Best brandy, two ounces.
(Dissolve the opium and the camphor first in the brandy.)
Syrup of ginger,
Syrup of lemon, of each sufficient to make six ounces.
Mix. Shake well.

Dose: For a child of one year or under, from four to six drops, in a little sweetened water; two years old, from eight to ten drops; four years old, twenty drops; adults, from one to one and one-half teaspoonfuls, from every half hour to four and six hours apart, as the case demands.

This is a sure cure for bloody flux, diarrhœa, and all relaxed conditions of the bowels. We never knew it to fail in a single case where there were no other complications. But, should there be inflammation of the bowels, you must put the patient on oat-meal water to drink and slippery elm, and injections of the same. Diet, extract of beef, milk punch, etc. See pages 14 and 17.

PILES—HEMORRHOIDS.

Fluid extract of hammamelis,
Fluid extract of ergot,
Fluid extract of hydrastis canadensis,
Fluid extract of collinsonia,
Fluid extract of pinus canadensis,
Tincture of arnica,
Tincture of laudanum,
Simple syrup,
Distilled water, of each one ounce.
Burnt alum, one-half drachm.
Glycerine of tannin, one-half ounce.
Mix.

Take a small ear syringe and inject ten or fifteen drops up into the rectum; after which lie down and keep quiet, and take a small tuft of pure cotton and saturate it with the mixture and keep it pressed up against the tumors, and keep them constantly moist with the medicine for several days, or longer if required. If the medicine is too strong for the inflamed parts, it can be weakened with a little sweet oil or simple syrup and oil. This will absorb the tumors in a very short 'time, as well as relieve the pain in this most distressing disease, and perform a cure in a very short time without resorting to surgical operations or caustics.

This is the most valuable remedy for this disease ever given to the world. The author has never failed to cure every case he has ever undertaken with this medicine. Ointments are useless, except the cosmoline.

INTERNAL REMEDY FOR HEMORRHOIDS.

Tincture of æsculas hipp., (horse-chestnut.)
Tincture of phytolacca decand, (poke-root) of each one-half ounce.
Mix.

Dose: Twenty drops in half a tumbler of water; teaspoonful every hour.

This should be taken for several days, mixing it up fresh every day in water.

COUGH SYRUPS.

There are so many kinds of coughs that arise from so many causes, we will proceed to give you a formula that you can always vary yourself to meet the indications. However, you must remember, that a syrup made from the spices, cloves, cinnamon, alspice, cardamon seed, etc., are always called for in a cough arising from no matter what cause. This you can make yourself and keep it on hand, and always add a little of this syrup to your cough syrup, just sufficient to flavor it. We will call this No. 1.

BALSAM FOR WEAK LUNGS—No. 2.

Oil of sweet almonds, one ounce.
Oil of anise, two drachms.
Gum Arabic, dissolved, one ounce.
Tincture of horehound, one ounce.
Tincture of Jamaica ginger, one-half ounce.
Syrup of stillingia, two ounces.
Syrup of honey, one ounce.
Good brandy, two ounces.
Mix.

Now you can add about one ounce of No. 1 to this, sufficient to make a ten-ounce mixture.

Dose: Half a teaspoonful every half hour till the cough is better, then prolong the intervals to one, two or three hours, as the case may require.

COUGHS FROM COLDS, WITH SORE LUNGS—No. 3.

Fluid extract of asclepias tub. (pleurisy root),
Fluid extract of sweet bugle weed (lycopus virg.),
Fluid extract of stone root (collinsonia), of each one drachm.
Tincture of lobelia seed, twenty drops.
Tincture of ipecac, one-half drachm.
Syrup of horehound, one ounce.
Syrup of stillingia, two ounces.
Good brandy, one ounce.
Mix.

Now you can add one-half ounce of No. 1.

Dose: Teaspoonful every hour or two hours; for children, reduce accordingly.

If either of these remedies are a little too strong they can always be reduced with a little water, or the juice of one lemon and water, to suit the requirements; and they all can be varied to suit the indications. Your druggist can put them up for you, and they will keep for years without spoiling.

Note.—The crab apple made into sauce is very good for all bronchial troubles, or you can stew and strain them, and add the juice to either of the above cough syrups, after sweetening to the taste. Now you have the finest cough medicines that we have ever used.

SPRAINS.

Take a large spoonful of honey, the same amount of salt and the white of one egg; beat the whole up incessantly for two hours; then let stand for one hour; then anoint the place sprained with the oil which will be produced from the mixture. This is said to have enabled persons with sprained ankles to walk, in twenty-four hours, entirely free from pain.—*King*.

HEALING SALVE.

One-half pound of beeswax, one-half pound of salty butter, one-quarter pound of turpentine, six ounces of the Balsam of Fir. Simmer slowly for half an hour, when it is ready for use.

Dr. Curtiss has used this preparation for years for old sores, wounds and burns, and has never found anything to surpass it.

Sure Cure for Bunions, or Frost-Bitten Feet.

Take the common glue, prepare it in the same way that the cabinet makers do, only pretty thick, spread it on a piece of linen the size you want it, and apply it to the bunion as hot as can be borne; let it remain there for several days, and repeat it if necessary. It will do it every time, for we have cured poor creatures many a time.

SCURVY.

Plenty of lemon juice, sweetened to taste, cures it every time, or lemon syrup or syrup of citric acid, may be used instead.

MISCELLANEOUS.

Tablespoonful of the juice of a roasted lemon, sweetened to the taste, is an excellent remedy for coughs, taken every two or three hours.

The juice of one lemon to a half a glass of water, sweetened just a little, used as a gargle, will cure many a mild case of diphtheria, and a little swallowed each time is all the better.

With the juice of two lemons added to a gill of water and one of brandy, and applied externally, we have cured many cases of erysipelas after all other remedies had failed.

The juice of one lemon, sweetened to taste, half a teaspoonful taken every fifteen minutes, has cured many a case of sick headache for us.

Lemonade is also an admirable drink for all kinds of cases of fevers.

It is also a grateful and refreshing drink for those who are well, when they are very tired and thirsty.

Equal parts of lemon juice and glycerine, will, ordinarily, remove tan and freckles from the face and hands. Try it.

RING WORM AND TETTER.

A strong tincture made from the green walnut hulls or rinds, and applied externally to the ring worm. Take half a pint of alcohol and add a handful of the green hulls to it, and let it stand for five or six days, is the way to get the tincture. Also, teaspoonful of this tincture added to a half tumbler of water; stir up well, and take a teaspoonful of this every hour internally. It is also advisable to take it for three or four days, making it fresh every morning.

ENLARGEMENT OF THE SPLEEN.

Fluid extract of grindelia squarrosa (new remedy),
Fluid extract of bearsfoot (Polymnia Uvedalia), of each one ounce·
Glycerine,
Distilled water, of each one ounce.
Mix.
Dose: Teaspoonful every three hours.
Get your druggist to put it up for you.

Good for the Kidneys in Dropsical Affections.

Bruised juniper berries,
Mustard seed,
Ginger, of each half ounce.
Bruised horse-radish,
Bruised parsley root, of each one ounce.
Old sour cider, one quart.
Let stand and infuse for several days.
Dose: Wineglass full three times per day.
This is excellent for kidney troubles.

HOW TO PREPARE POULTICES.

Equal parts of ground flax seed, slippery elm bark and oat meal, for general purposes, is the best kind of a poultice that we have ever used. It can be mixed with either hot or cold water, as desired for the occasion. If the surface is very tender, it is better to be warm than cold when applied. It should be well mixed, that there are no lumps in it; not too thin nor too thick. This poultice will keep moist longer than either of the above ingredients by itself. This is the way we always prescribe our poultices; however, they are mostly made from either one of the above articles.

BREAD POULTICE.

Take several slices of bread, pour over them sufficient hot water, and let stand for an hour or so, that the bread may be soft; then pour off the water, and with a fork beat the bread up into a thick dough; spread this on a piece of linen previously cut the size you wish it. Bread poultices are very valuable for their bland effect for all irritating surfaces.

For gangreenous and bad smelling ulcers or sores of any kind, sprinkle some pulverized charcoal over the ulcer before applying the poultice, and it can also be mixed with the poultice. Charcoal poultices correct offensive smells from foul sores, and favor a healthy action.

Poultices are chiefly used in the following complaints: Pneumonia, pleurisy, bronchitis, peritonitis, acute rheumatism, lumbago, and to mature and facilitate the discharges of matter in abcesses, boils, etc. When used to mature abscesses or disperse inflammation, poultices should always extend beyond the surface of the inflamed tissues, but after the inflammation is subdued and the abscess is discharging, the poultice should not be much larger than to just cover the opening through which the matter is escaping; if continued too large, they irritate, and may develop other boils or abscesses around the old one. Poultices over the chest or abdomen should be made very thick and not too thin, as they dry very soon. They must be well secured by suitable jackets or bandages sufficient to hold them in place. They should be often changed on those parts, but do not disturb the old one till the new one is all ready to replace it.

Poultices can be made from many different kinds of substances that may have valuable medicinal properties.

POTATO POULTICE.

Boil the common potato in the usual way, mash them and mix them with ground elm bark. This is a valuable poultice for acute inflammatory sore eyes, applied very thin and changed often. Also, the raw scraped potato, in the shape of a poultice, is very valuable for the same purpose.

MUSTARD POULTICE.

If you wish a very quick action from this poultice, mix the mustard with vinegar alone into a thick paste, spread it on the cloth thin with a case-knife as you would butter on your bread, and lay it on the affected parts next to the skin. It will take effect in a very few minutes. You can oil the skin just a little, and as the mustard dries it will not stick to the skin or annoy your patient. This is the way it should always be applied to the soles of the feet, if you expect any benefit from it, and changed often before it gets dry. But if you wish it to work slower, you can mix it with equal parts of vinegar and water, and add a little wheat flour to the mustard; spread on your cloth a little thicker than the other way; then lay a very thin piece of linen over the mustard before you apply the poultice to the patient. A mustard poultice should be kept on from ten to twenty minutes at least, till the skin is drawn very red and is irritable afterwards. It is said that if the white of an egg is mixed with the mustard it will never draw into a blister, and thus it can be kept on longer, which is very beneficial.

HOW TO MAKE FOMENTATIONS.

Fomentations are employed for the purpose of lessening pain and inflammation, and for relaxing the parts. They are usually composed of bitter herbs, steeped for a time in hot water or vinegar and water, and then placed in muslin, cloth or sacks and applied over the affected parts as hot as can be borne. Care should be taken not to moisten or stain the patient's clothes or the bed. They are to be removed often and changed for new hot ones; if the pain or inflammation is severe, the oftener they should be changed for hot ones.

Hop and vinegar fomentations are very valuable for pain in the head, bowels, or any other parts of the body.

St. Johnswort or the poke-root are very valuable, applied hot to the mammary breasts, to disperse or scatter the inflammatory condition, caked breasts or tumors and swellings; or the wild indigo fomentation is valuable for dispelling tumors from the breasts. The smartweed is also good.

The Mullein fomentation surpasses everything else that we know of for dispelling bruises or swellings in man or beast. A strong decoction made from the mullein leaves, applied, hot or cold, to sprains, bruises or swellings, is the best remedy that we know of at present. We have used it for years, on both man and beast, with the most astonishing results.

VALUABLE TOOTH WASH.

Gum guaiacum,
Orris root, of each, one ounce;
Camphor gum, one drachm.

Put these ingredients in a pint of good brandy; let the mixture infuse for ten days, shaking it occasionally; then strain the mixture through a cotton cloth into a clean bottle.

Wash and cleanse the teeth once in twenty-four hours with this preparation, and bleeding, enlarged or detached gums will be healed, lessened and restored in their proper place, and the tooth-ache will seldom be experienced. This is the most valuable preparation we have ever used.

TOOTH-ACHE.

For immediate relief for this dreadful affliction, take
Oil of cloves,
Oil of cinnamon,
Creosote, of each, half drachm;
Chloroform, half ounce.
Mix.

Take a tuft of cotton wound around the end of a little stick; now saturate the cotton in the mixture, and bathe the gum on each side of the tooth with the medicine. If the tooth has a cavity in it, put a piece of cotton, saturated with the medicine, in the cavity. This will smart and burn for a little while, but no matter; it will cure the tooth-ache for the time.

Poisons and their Antidotes.

Nothing that appertains to domestic treatment is of greater value than a knowledge of poisons and the treatment necessary in cases of accidental or premeditated poisoning. So many substances of a poisonous nature are used in manufactures, among farmers and mechanics, and also in private houses, that it will be useful to have a guide to refer to in case of accident, for in almost every case of poisoning the antidote must be instantly given or else success cannot be expected.

As a general rule, in all cases of poisoning, especially if seen immediately after the poison is swallowed, the indication is to make the person *vomit*. To bring this about, give a teaspoonful of mustard in a tumbler of water, or two or three teaspoonfuls of powdered alum in the same way. *Vomiting* can in all cases be promoted by tickling the throat with a feather.

ARSENIC.

Articles: Scheele's green, arsenious acid, arpiment, King's yellow, realgar, fly powder, arsenical paste and soap, rat poison.

Symptoms.—Pain and burning in the stomach, dryness of throat, cramps, purging, vomiting, hoarseness and difficulty of speech, eyes red and sparkling, suppression of urine, matter vomited greenish or yellowish.

Treatment.—Give large quantities of milk and raw eggs, limewater, or flour and water. Then castor oil, or if tincture of iron is within reach, take from half to a full teaspoonful of it, and mix with it a little bi-carbonate of soda or saleratus, and administer it to the person, and follow it with an emetic. This acts as a real antidote—the chemical combination resulting being insoluble in the fluids of the stomach.

COPPER.

Articles.—Blue copperas, blue verditer, mineral green, verdigris, food cooked in copper vessels, pickles made green by copper.

Symptoms.—Coppery taste in the mouth, tongue dry and parched, very painful colic, bloody stools, convulsions.

Treatment.—Large quanties of milk and white of eggs, afterwards strong tea. *Vinegar should not be given.*

IRON.

Articles.—Sulphate of iron (copperas), green vitriol, chloride of iron.

Symptoms.—Colic pains, constant vomiting and purging, violent pain in throat, coldness of skin, feeble pulse.

Treatment.—Give an emetic, afterwards magnesia or carbonate of soda and water; also mucilaginous drinks.

LEAD.

ARTICLES.—Acetate or sugar of lead, white lead, red lead, litharge.

SYMPTOMS.—Metallic taste in mouth, pain in stomach and bowels, painful vomiting—often blood, hiccough. If taken for some time, obstinate colic, paralysis—partial or complete, obstinate constipation, diminution of urine.

TREATMENT.—Put two ounces of epsom salts into a pint of water and give a wineglassful every ten minutes until it operates freely.

PHOSPHORUS.

ARTICLE.—Lucifer matches.

SYMPTOMS—Pain in stomach and bowels, vomiting, diarrhea, tenderness and tension of the abdomen, great excitement of the whole system.

TREATMENT.—Prompt emetic, copious draughts of warm water containing magnesia, chalk, whiting or even flour. *No oils or fat should be given.*

OPIUM.

ARTICLES.—Laudanum, paregoric, black drop, soothing syrups, cordials, syrup of poppies, morphine, Dover's powder, etc.

SYMPTOMS.—Giddiness, stupor—gradually increasing to a deep sleep, pupil of the eyes very small, lips blue, skin cold, heavy, slow breathing.

TREATMENT.—Make the patient vomit as quickly as possible. Use mustard and warm water or salt and water, and tickle the throat with a feather. After vomiting, give plenty of coffee, and place a mustard poultice around the calf of each leg, and, if the patient is cold and sinking, give stimulants and rouse him to walking or running by your assistance. Beat the soles of his feet, dash cold water on the face, and do anything to prevent him from sleeping until the effects have passed off, for if he goes to sleep it is the sleep of death.

STRYCHNINE.

ARTICLES.—Rat poison, nux vomica, St. Ignatius bean.

SYMPTOMS.—Lockjaw, twitching of the muscles, convulsions, the body is bent backwards so as to rest on the feet and head only.

TREATMENT.—Empty the stomach by an emetic, then give linseed tea or barley water, and to an adult give thirty drops of laudanum, to relieve the spasms. A teaspoonful of ether can also be given.

OTHER POISONOUS PLANTS OR SEEDS.

Such as false mushrooms, belladonna, henbane, or anything a child may have eaten, or taken in mistake by any person. Vegetable poisons act either as an irritant, acro-narcotic or narcotic. If it is an irritant, the symptoms are an acrid, pungent taste, with more or less bitterness, excessive heat, great dryness of the mouth and throat, with a sense of tightness there, violent vomiting, purging, with great pain in the stomach and bowels, breathing often quick and difficult, appearance of intoxication, eye frequently dilated, insensibility, resembling death. The symptoms of narcotic poisons are described under Opium.

TREATMENT.—If an irritant, and vomiting does occur and continues, render it easier by large draughts of warm water, but if symptoms of insensibility have come on without vomiting, empty the stomach with any emetic that may be at hand, and after the operation of the emetic, give a sharp purgative. After as much as is possible of the poison is got rid of, very strong black coffee, or vinegar diluted with water, may be given with advantage. Camphor mixture with a little ether may be frequently given, and if insensibility is considerable, warmth and frictions may be employed.

Rules to Administer Medicines.

Suppose the dose for an adult to be one drachm:

A child under	1 year	will require but	one-twelfth,	or 5 grains;
"	2 years	"	one-eighth,	or 8 grains;
"	3 years	"	one-sixth,	or 10 grains;
"	4 years	"	one-quarter,	or 15 grains;
"	7 years	"	one-third,	or 1 scruple;
"	13 years	"	one-half,	or ½ drachm;
"	20 years	"	two-thirds,	or 2 scruples;

A person above 21 years, the full dose of one drachm.
A person of 75, the inverse gradation of the above.

This is an excellent table for regulating the doses of medicines. A mixture, powder, pill, or draught, may be proportioned to a nicety by attention to the above rules.

To Measure Medicine Instead of Weighing.

A drachm of any substance that is near the weight of water, will fill a common teaspoon level full. Four teaspoonfuls make a tablespoonful, or one-half of an ounce. Two tablespoonfuls, an ounce, and so on. On the same principle, one-third of a teaspoonful will be one scruple, or twenty grains in weight.

Doses Varied According to Age.

The doses of medicines recommended for an adult, or grown person, may be varied to the age of the patient, according to the following rule:

Two-thirds of the dose for a person from fourteen to sixteen;
One-half " " seven to ten;
One-third " " four to six;
One-fourth " " three years old;
One-eighth " " one year old.

LIQUID MEASURE.

A tablespoonful contains half an ounce;
A pint " sixteen ounces;
A teacup " one gill;
A wineglass " two ounces;
A teaspoonful " sixty drops;
Four teaspoonfuls are equal to one tablespoonful.

DRY MEASURE.

A tablespoonful contains four drachms, or half an ounce;
A teaspoonful " one drachm;
A teaspoonful " sixty grains.

DOSES OF MEDICINE.

The following scale has been established for the regulation of the doses of medicine in general.

If the dose for a person of middle age be one drachm, the dose for one from fourteen to twenty-one years of age will be two scruples, or two-thirds as much.

From seven to fourteen, half a drachm, or one-half.

From four to seven, one scruple, or one-third.

The dose for a child of four years will be fifteen grains, or one-quarter.

For a child three years old, ten grains, or half a scruple.

For one two years old, eight grains.

For one a year old, five grains, or one-twelfth as much as for a person of middle age.

Women, in general, require smaller doses than men, owing to a difference in size and constitution.

Since the Fluid Extracts and Specific Tinctures have been introduced, of course the doses are all much smaller than the above table, but they are of the same ratio as the above scale.

General Remarks.

The reader of our little book will see that we have not gone into any description whatever of medicinal plants—as is usually done in all other domestic medical works—for the reason you will see more fully explained in an article on the Progress of Medicine, given at the close of our book, which we desire you to read over carefully. But, instead, we have given you our Prescriptions, just as we would write you one should you come to see us in person, and send you to the drug store to get the fluid extracts and mother tinctures which are now made from the roots and herbs gathered in their proper season. The sciences of Botany and Chemistry have taught us how to extract the active medicinal principles from these plants; therefore the manufacturing scientists, who are responsible parties, have now men of science and experience constantly employed gathering these medicinal plants from all over the country, the result of which is that, within the last three or four years, the scientific pharmacies have given to the world a universal standard strength from the active medicinal principles of the medicinal plants. This is a great achievement, a triumph which we have never known before. This fact gives to the physician, as well as to the common people, the advantage of procuring, at any of the first-class druggists, a pure article of the active principle of any kind of drug which we want. No matter where obtained, you can rely upon it as a universal standard of strength. These drugs are in the shape of fluid extracts, specific tinctures, the sulphates, resinoids, and alcoloids.

This is very desirable from the fact that it makes the dose so small and so much more agreeable to the taste, the dose now being only drops and grains and fractions of a grain, and from a half drachm to a drachm, and far more reliable in its effect. Those are facts which are certainly very desirable for us to know, when we consider that only a few years ago, when we were in the night of our ignorance, we had to gather the plants regardless of their season, and boil and stew them to make teas and decoctions which were of the crude material, and pour down the throats of the patients whole teacupfuls, and in many cases a pint and over, for a dose of those crude drugs. Then we were ignorant of the fact that the stomach and human system have to be their own chemical laboratory, out of which this pint dose of medicine after a great deal of labor on the part of the stomach, could only extract about half a drop of the active principle of the drug, the balance being wholly waste material that the human system must labor to get rid of.

Hence our little book is a timely messenger—Pearls of Wisdom. Gems of Knowledge—that you all may know that you need not, must not, buy any more roots and herbs at a drug store, thinking to make your own medicine, for you can't do it; besides, many of these crude drugs have been lying in the stores for years, all worm-eaten and dusty, and as worthless as a handful of chips gathered from an old wood-pile, while the active principles of the drug made from the green root gathered in its proper season and manufactured into fluid extract, tincture, etc., will keep for years in well stopped bottles, at the end of which time they are perfectly safe and reliable. Hence you can see that if we have a universal standard of strength agreed upon by the scientific pharmacists, then we are safe, since the only competition will consist in the different manufacturing houses to see which can outdo the other in furnishing to the world from this agreed standard of strength a purer article of drugs, more palatable, and therefore more desirable.

This, dear reader, is the reason that we have said nothing about the medicinal plants in our book. This is the reason that we have given you our Prescriptions as we have, and directed you to go to your druggist to have them filled. The cost of these prescriptions in many instances will be much higher than the medicine used to cost you, on account of their purity. However, what you pay now in the cost of your medicines you will more than save in the quality, as much less in quantity is now required.

The History and Origin of Medicine.

Medicine is, no doubt, coeval with the history of human suffering, but as a profession, it first began in the early accounts given of the Egyptians. The priests of the early nations were the practitioners of the healing art, but from all accounts they were exceedingly empirical, making use of but few remedies, the most of which were external applications, together with incantations and ceremonies to affect the imagination, though their efficiency in curing disease was, for the most part, due to their knowledge of a few medicinal principles.

Hippocrates was the first to arrange the principles of medicine into an attempted science, while Aesculapius first made it an exclusive study and practice. Aesculapius flourished about twelve hundred and fifty years before Christ; his two sons became celebrated as surgeons in the Greek armies during the Trojan war.

Fifty years after the destruction of Troy, a temple was built in honor to Aesculapius, who was then worshiped as one of the gods.

The worship of this god soon spread throughout all Greece and passed into Asia, Africa and Italy, so that multitudes of temples were erected in honor to his name, and in which he was worshiped.

These temples were erected in the midst of the most delightful scenery, and statutes of colossal proportions were erected to represent the god of medicine.

Pythagoras first introduced the practice of visiting patients at their homes: (500 years B. C.) He rejected all theories in medicine, and contended that experience was the only safe guide to a successful practice.

About three hundred years before Christ, Ptolemy founded a medical school in Alexandria in Egypt, and among the Ptolemies the most celebrated were Erasistratus and Herophilus, who were the first to dissect the dead. These men opposed blood-letting and the use of all violent remedies and trusted to nature in the cure of disease. They paid particular attention to the action of the heart, and were the first to observe the pulse and its variations.

The Pythagoreans became the dominant school, partly through the earnest efforts of Hippocrates (430 years B. C.) who opened up an earnest warfare upon the superstitious ceremonies of the Aesculapian priests, though he, in his practice, still adhered to bleeding and purging.

Three hundred and twenty years before Christ, the Alexandrian library was formed, which had a happy effect upon the departments of medicine, anatomy and physiology. In this library there were 600,000 volumes or rolls which contained all the valuable information of previous ages.

One hundred and thirty years after Christ, Galen was born in Pergamos, and 500 years after his birth, the Alexandrian library was burned by Caliph Omar. Galen had access to this library; he traveled much and wrote largely on subjects connected with medicine. He was an independent thinker and paid but little heed to what was then called authority. So great was his learning and wisdom that he obtained the reputation of "cracle." He thoroughly studied all the schools of medicine and philosophy, and then selected from all, except from the Epicurians, which he totally rejected. Galen determined to gather from the various sources all that was useful in the treatment of disease. He was, perhaps, the first "eclectic" in the practice of medicine.

From the twelfth to the fifteenth century, the practice of medicine was again confined chiefly to the priests, who were men of learning and who became the principal physicians.

About this time an attempt to investigation was made by a class of men who seemed to think that, while physical science was making some gigantic strides, there was no reason why medical science should be so comparatively slow, but a large majority believed that no progress was possible and hence, to shield their ignorance, they attacked every species of investigation in the most vehement manner, which in the least conflicted with their narrow and illiberal views.

In 1628, Harvey discovered the circulation of the blood, for which he was called the "circulator." in derision. He was deprived of the right to practice medicine, and was threatened with banishment. He was finally compelled to leave his native country, to escape the obloquy heaped upon him, and he finally died without seeing the benefits of his investigations.

In 1638, the wife of an ex-king of Peru was persuaded, while suffering with a malarial fever, to try the cinchona, and was afterwards restored to health. Ten years after, a Jesuit endeavored to introduce the Peruvian bark in Europe, and he was denounced as a quack, and the common people were persuaded to believe that the bark created disease instead of curing it.

PRESENT MEDICAL SCHOOLS.

The different philosophies of ancient times have given rise to different theories, and hence in our times we have different medical schools, each of which base their practice upon the peculiar philosophy they have adopted. It will not be out of place now to give a short description of the peculiar features of the medical schools of the present day. Of these, we have the Allopathic, Homeopathic, and Eclectic as the chief, while there are some minor schools, as the Botanic and Hydropathic.

THE ALLOPATHIC SCHOOL.

This school of medicine comprises a large class of the physicians of the present day. They are known among the common people as "old school doctors," "mineral doctors," "calomel doctors," "allopaths," and "regulars." They are justly entitled to the term "old school," for their present treatment does not materially differ from that of Hyppocrates, who flourished twenty-two centuries ago.

They base their theory of practice upon the Latin maxim, "Contraria Contrarius Curanter," which implies that disease must be cured by antagonism—that if a person has a disease, another disease should be set up in the system, contrary to the one already there, and in this way they attempt to modify diseased conditions. For this, they frequently gave calomel to salivate the system, and by this salivation they expected to counteract the already existing disease. Later years, however, many of this school have modified their views upon this subject, and hence they endeavor to avoid the force of their Latin motto.

Though at first they gloried in the name of Allopathic, many of them now despise the name, on account of the force of its meaning Allopathic is from the Greek, *allos*—other, and *pathos*—disease; other disease), and hence they choose to be known by the somewhat exclusive title of "regulars."

While there is a modification in these respects, there is a disposition to adhere to the old landmarks, and hence the philosophy remains the same; but their practice seems to be gradually leaving the old paths. The Allopathic profession of to-day is not what it was forty years ago in many respects. A very large class of this school are in favor of progress and improvement, and in keeping up with the times, while others seem to think profession should be stereotyped into a general routine.

This school gives medicine in sensible doses and pays but little attention to the taste. Their medicines for the most part are drastic and powerful, on which account much objection has been raised by the weakly and delicate.

BOTANICAL SCHOOL.

It will be needless to say much here concerning this system of practice, as it is now almost extinct. The physicians of this school are known as "vegetable doctors," "root doctors," "herb doctors," "Indian doctors," "steam doctors," "botanics," "Thompsonians," and, of later times, "physiopaths." Dr. Thompson started out with an utter disgust for the old methods of practice. He inveighed against the use of minerals, and chose the vegetable kingdom as his field for medicinal agents. Some good has been accomplished by Thompson and his followers, but the system never rose from its nudity. Thompson himself was quite illiterate, and the system was crude and could not bear the tests of a sound philosophy. Its method of curing disease was by severe drenching, with hot and nauseating teas, made from the common roots and herbs. The system never arose to a very high state of respectability, which, in part, was owing to its proscriptive principles and its severe method of treating disease.

HOMEOPATHIC SCHOOL.

Owing much to the objectionable features in Allopathy, a new system arose upon a philosophy advocated by Hahneman, the Latin term of which is "Similia Similitus Curanter," by which they mean that medicines which produce upon the healthy subject certain diseased conditions, are also capable of curing similar diseases as they arise spontaneously. They claim that "the medicine sets up in the suffering part of the organization an artificial, but somewhat stronger, disease, which, on account of its great similarity and preponderating influence, takes the place of the former, and the organism from that time forth is affected only by the artificial complaint. This, from the minute doses of medicine, soon subsides and leaves the patient altogether free from disease."

A person in reading this might suppose that the differences between the above two schools were but slight; but there is a vast difference and a great gulf fixed between them. The Allopath would think it beneath his dignity to counsel with a Homeopath, and this the Homeopath seems to care but little about, while he flatters himself to be the most successful of the two.

The minute doses of medicine in the Homeopathic practice are made by diluting or attenuating their drugs in a systematic way so as to decrease their potency in a geometrical manner. Their medicines do not differ from the Allopathic so much in kind as they do in amount and manner of preparing. They aim to please the palate, which is certainly a commendable feature, when it can be done without sacrificing the disease for the taste. For instance, where the Allopath would give ten grains of calomel, the Homeopath would take but one grain of the drug, and to this he would add sugar of milk and make a thousand doses. He sometimes gives a millionth or a quintillionth part of a grain or drop. Here, then, is a great difference. Their method of trituration is to take one grain of medicine and mix it with ninety-nine grains of sugar of milk; this is put into a bottle and marked one hundredth. To prepare the second degree, one grain of the one hundredth is triturated with ninety-nine grains of sugar of milk, and this constitutes the one ten-thousanth. The third potency is formed by taking one grain of the one ten-thousandth and triturating with ninety-nine grains of sugar of milk, which constitutes one millionth. These are called first, second and third potencies. Thus they continue, always taking one grain of the last trituration and mixing it with ninety-nine grains of sugar of milk, until they get down to the five-thousandth potency. The liquids or tinctures are treated in a similar manner, though drops are used instead of grains, and alcohol is used instead of sugar of milk.

There is much difference of opinion among the homeopaths in the use of their potencies. Some use the 1st, 2d and 3d potencies, while others practice with their 30th, and others contend for the 200th, while a fourth class declare better results in the use of the 500th.

While some things in homeopathy may appear quite vague and ethereal, as a general thing there is to be found quite a liberal and progressive spirit amongst them, and hence they have a wide range of medicinal agents, and some of the late discoveries in medicine are due to the progressive spirit of homeopathy.

There is no denying the fact that too much strong medicine has been used in former days, and we should hail with delight that spirit which has for its object the improvement of medical science.

ECLECTIC SCHOOL.

We cannot describe this school any better than Dr. Yankin of St. Louis, has. He says:

"The Eclectics are becoming quite a popular class of medical practitioners. They have at this day a bright galaxy of scholars, philosophers and philanthropists, who are devoting themselves with zeal and industry worthy of all praise to the study and practice of medicine and surgery. Their colleges of learning are becoming somewhat numerous, and their written volumes on the different branches of medical science, adorn the libraries of almost all physicians of the different schools. Theirs is a science made up by an inductive system of reasoning. They have added to their store-house of knowledge, by an earnest study of all the various systems, and selecting such agents as have been proven good and useful in whatever school they could be found. In taking their survey, they saw much to be condemned and much to be commended in all the schools of medicine, hence they chose to found a new basis of medical practice in which should be incorporated the good of all schools, while the bad should be rejected. They belong to the progressive class, and claim that none should be so bound up in theories as not to receive truth wherever found, whether

'In christian lands or on heathen grounds.'

They combine the sweetness of homeopathy with all that is good in allopathy, hydropathy, or botanic practice, as well as many discoveries of their own. Their progress for the last fifteen years has been surprisingly great, so much so that even their old standard authors are claimed to be behind the times. Their present mode of treating disease is very nearly as pleasant as in homeopathy, and they claim that the power of their agents will reach the disease more readily, and cure the patient in a much shorter time than either of the two former schools. The per cent. or death-rate is claimed not to be as great as found in the statistics of other schools.

On account of the sound of the word ECLECTIC, some of the common people have thought that it had something to do with electricity, but this is not the case. They use electricity as they use any other agent, but they do not use it as their exclusive right. ECLECTIC means SELECT. They aim to select the best of all.

The medicines they employ in the treatment of disease, are such agents as will restore the healthy action of all the organs of the human body. They endeavor to avoid the violent and irritating drugs, believing that they tend to produce disease and prostrate the system. They seek to support the system and not to depress it. They nourish their patients instead of starving them. They aim to restore the healthy action of the liver, kidneys, stomach, and intestines, by assisting nature to throw off diseased action.

Eclecticism has for its basis the laws of physiology and hygiene. It enjoins upon its practitioners a careful study of all the functions of the body, and teaches that disease is a departure from healthy action, produced either by "excess, defect or perversion."

To relieve a patient from disease, they teach that the first thing is to know what the symptoms are, and their cause; secondly, to have a thorough knowledge of the effects of remedies, and just what drug is specially indicated in the individual case; the latter of which is obtained by a thorough study of all the materia medica taught by the different schools of medicine.

They use counter irritants, but they seldom blister; they use opiates to relieve pain, but they do not depend upon them as means of cure; they use but few drugs that cannot be readily eliminated from the system.

We have no doubt but that there has been more *progress* in medical science within the last ten years than within the last hundred years. More especially has this been in the direction of furnishing to the world a purer article of medicines—fluid extracts, specific tinctures, resinoids, alcaloids, etc., the active principles from all medicinal substances—and with it has come to us a better knowledge of how to employ them than was ever known before. Therefore, it will be appropriate for us to note the fact, first, that in all domestic medical books for the use of families, the crude remedies, roots and herbs, prepared in decoctions, or teas, have been recommended, to which we have serious objections, which we will proceed to explain and make plain to our readers.

Through the aid of chemical science, we have learned that the medicinal properties of a plant, which of course means to any part of the plant which is to be used, depends entirely upon the time in the season—we mean the time in the year—when it is gathered, when it is known by experience the healing properties are best. Then, again, the healing properties are subjected to the contingencies of the season. We will endeavor to illustrate our meaning. If, for instance, the best time for gathering a plant is in the month of September, then this statement is made in the sense that the season has been of the most favorable condition for producing the healthiest properties of the plant (for plants can be sickly, you know), for if the season has been more dry than usual, or more wet than common, it will be perceived at a glance that the remedy gathered one year will be of an entirely different strength than the same remedy gathered in another year, or in a different locality, country and soil. Hence they cannot be made reliable if you should make them into decoctions or teas. Therefore, it has been the aim of our great modern chemists and observers and pioneers to give to the world a system of remedial agents that will be uniform; that is, all manufacturers shall give to the world the solid or fluid extracts, specific tinctures, resinoids and alcaloids all of equal strength, and at all times, which can be relied upon; that if the dose of the remedy be that of ten drops to produce its medicinal effect, that it will be the same all over the world; also, that the same dose shall produce the medicinal effect next year as it did this year. Hence, our experience and our confidence has led us to rely upon the tinctures, fluid extracts, alcaloids, etc., etc., which the leading manfacturers in the United States have furnished us. Our manufacturers of these botanical remedies have carried off the palm of excellence and superiority everywhere that they have been placed in competition with the celebrated manufacturers of Europe at all the great international exhibitions of our day.

These are the reasons why we have advised you all through our book to get your druggist to fill your prescriptions for you. Copy them off, or, better still, take your book to the druggist and show him which prescription you want filled, then you need fear no mistake. In this sense our book is new and in its style entirely original with ourselves. Therefore we commend this reasoning to the common sense and good judgment of our readers.

In the early days of medical progress in this country, the eminent Dr. Warren, who founded the first Alopathic college in the city of Boston, in one of his medical books, in the most beautiful language has paid the highest tribute to the Eclectic school of medicine that we have ever heard. We feel that our little book would not be complete without giving you some extracts taken from his book, which was published in 1858. He says:

"There is a large and growing class of physicians, called at first, after the founder of the school, Thomsonian. Subsequently they were known as the Botanic physicians, and now pass under the title of Eclectics. These men, directing their attention at first chiefly to the Cayenne and the Lobelia, have greatly extended their zealous researches over the vegetable kingdom, and have gathered much information worthy to be preserved. These researches have revealed a sadly neglected duty on the part of the old school practitioners, and in 1852 drew from the Committee on Indigenous Medicinal Botany, appointed by the American Medical Association, the confession that our practitioners generally have been extremely ignorant of the medicinal plants even in their own neighborhoods, and to this fact the committee attribute it that the Eclectic physicians had in many cases supplanted the Regulars in the confidence of the people. The education and talent of this class of practitioners have gradually risen year by year, till at the present time they have several medical schools, where students are well instructed by men of real ability. The vast list of valuable remedies that these men have given to the world, drawn wholly from our home plants, are a boon of no small value. I regard them as equal in value to all that we were previously in possession of. And yet it is very mortifying that the remedies which these men have given us are by hundreds of our old school practitioners not even known by name, and even where they are known, generally not honored with a trial. 'King's American Dispensatory,' a book of 1,800 pages, in which these plants are well described, is almost unknown among us. Aside from a copy in my own library, I do not know that one is owned by any other member of the Massachusetts Medical Society. However learned a man may be, he is not fully equipped as a practitioner without his full acquaintance with this class of medicines."

[We will add that this valuable book, King's Dispensatory, is not owned nor known much about by one in a hundred old-school practitioners, even at this late date, 1880.]

"But all are useful in a degree. On the whole, I am disposed to regard all the operators and provers in the different departments of medicine as very useful in a degree, no matter to what school they belong, or what class of men, except, always, those mercenary quacks who lie about their remedies to make money. But each of all those sincere and honest men who believe what they teach, is aiding in some measure the general advancement of science. Although the truths, as they present them, are but fragmentary, they may prove useful in the hands of the true, liberal and progressive men who have chosen for themselves the name and title of Eclectics, which means all those men who have the wisdom as well as the independence to select the best things out of all systems of medicine. And that brings us to the remark that the general conclusion must be that there is but one truly liberal and philosophical school of medicine, and that is the Eclectic, composed of that class of thinking men who have liberality enough, as well as independence, to reject all and every exclusive system of medicine, and receive out of all systems only those things which are approved by experience and reason.

PROGRESS OF MEDICINE.

There have been long periods when the science and art of healing made scarcely any progress; but now they are advancing, and in some departments quite fast. The chemistry in man—commonly called animal chemistry—has opened up many sources of light which in the past were unknown. And but very few physicians have yet commenced the study of these very essential branches of medical science; but the delinquents are but sleeping in the rear of this rapid advance, and will soon awaken to find themselves among the ghosts of a dead generation.

Liebig, a distinguished student in chemistry, has made many very valuable discoveries to open the way for inquiry into this department. Simons, also, has perhaps done more. Mealhe is exploring still deeper, and has made valuable discoveries, of which the students in medicine will have these problems before their minds, bye and bye, and they will be compelled to answer them and govern their actions upon them as well—inquiries and propositions like the following:

What are the chemical compositions of the solids and fluids of the human body?

What is the nature of the changes which occur in the composition of the solids and fluids during disease?

What alterations in the chemical compositions of the solids and fluids take place during the operations of medicine before it can exert any remote action on the animal economy?

A remedy must be absorbed, and before it can be absorbed, ti must be soluble in the fluids of the human body.

Medicines are subject to chemical changes during their passage through the system.

Those changes are regulated by ordinary chemical law, and may, therefore, to some extent, be protected and made available in the cure of disease. And then, again, those laws are disturbed and varied to some extent by the law of vitality; just as the needle is disturbed and made to vary by disturbing forces.

What are those disturbances, and to what extent and under what circumstances do they occur? With those and similar inquiries and propositions before the intelligent physician's mind, diligently studied, the physician will learn, in time, to prescribe with some intelligent aim.

He will not know everything, to be sure, but what he does know, he will have a rational reason for knowing.

If he gives a medicine with these facts before him, he will have in view the chemical changes of the solids and fluids of the body known to be disturbed by disease, which he is trying to combat.

He will, at the same time, try to keep in mind the solution of medicine in the fluids of the body, as well as the chemical reactions between the component parts and the acids and alkalies, etc., found in the alimentary tubes and elsewhere.

As the science of medicine advances and becomes progressive in its march and eclectic in its character, gathering from all systems the best attested facts, and learning to use them to the exclusion of all systems of mere theories, and liberal sufficient only to hold the present facts in subordination to future experience, then, and not till then, will the medical profession be progressive. With such men as these, the science of medicine will advance, and the light of to-morrow will then be modified by the light of to-day. Such men as these will everywhere be found knocking at the door for admission into some new department of Nature.

NEED OF LIBERALITY.

The medical profession, to be real physicians, must be free from bigotry; they must have no narrow prejudice against any man or class of men, but be always ready to examine carefully and candidly any new remedy that is brought to their notice, from no matter what source it may come. They must not hedge themselves about with such restrictive by-laws and society rule as are calculated to fetter their thoughts; that will turn their investigations by a sort of moral necessity into the narrow channels of mere party conservatism.

Remember, that he that is once enclosed by such restrictions must hew a path for his feet through bigotry and malevolence itself, before he can escape them, or be a free man in any noble sense. When the professors of the healing art can hoard medical knowledge as misers hoard gold, and can submit its purity to equally certain tests, then it will be time and appear in better taste for them to grow exclusive. Until then the most becoming badge that they can wear would be that of the Christian adage, "let each esteem others better than himself."

MEDICAL SCIENCE,

With liberal by-laws, is fitted to do a great deal of good. But it will be hard to show that those with stringently restrictive rules can operate otherwise than as a check upon progress. In truth, they are apt to become mere catacombs in which only to embalm dead ideas of the past. They are liable to become the instruments for accomplishing the ambition of a few leading, narrow, conservative men with brainless heads, who attempt to suppress everything of a progressive nature which should happen to be outside of their organization, and they beget a feeling like that which would forbid the fixed stars from shedding a drop of their light into our atmosphere, without first coming down and joining the solar system.

CONSERVATIVE LEADERS.

There is no influence which holds so steady a check upon medical progress as those conservative leaders in many of our medical associations; not that they are opposed to any improvement in medical art, nor would they object to any amount of discovery if it would only come to the profession through channels which they have the honor of opening, but against all light from outside or from obscure sources they will draw down the curtain and close the doors; and if it should chance to get within their sacred enclosure, they will call it darkness, and the priests of the temple to atone for the indignity offered to the gods of medicine, and fill the whole sky with murky clouds from their altars. Those men have strong faith in cast; therefore, in low places of society, they look for nothing but ignorance and poverty, notwithstanding the light of every natural day breaks in the horizon and ascends. They so far despise analogies as to insist that all medical light breaks at what they call the zenith of the profession, and comes down. With them the temples of Esculapius are all rebuilt and they are the priests, and, therefore, to offer in sacrifice the smallest part of a medical plant is sacrilege, unless it be intrusted to their hands. Those are the men who regard knowledge as a contraband article, unless regularly entered at the custom house, with bills of lading properly certified to by the conservative magnates at some other metropolis. With them knowledge is not like the west wind, fanning the brow of the peasant as gently as that of a king; not like the bright light of heaven, entering the small, clean window of the hut as readily as the large one of the palace; not as a boon, which comes alike freely to all; and which is to be everywhere amplified, changed as circumstances and conditions require, and adapted to the present hour. We would not be unjust or severe, but we cannot but remark further, that these men present but one view to humanity—they are monotonous objects of inspection. Look at them a thousand times, and you see but the same unaltered phase of life.

And to the mariner on life's ocean they are not safe lights to go by, for if he approaches them on the dark side they remain just as black as night, unless he should come around to their shining front. They are not revolving lights; they have lights, to be sure, and may be bright and genial, but it only gleams out upon the waters in one direction; it does not sweep around and throw its direct rays upon every mariner's path. Such men as these can only be useful to a few and a certain class. They have in them no true omniology; they are not all-teaching; their lives are not all-instructive, only to their friends, their clique or party, or school. They have length, but not breadth. They are citizens of Boston, New York, Philadelphia or Cincinnati; but not of the world.

THE TRUE PHYSICIAN.

How different the character of a true man or a physician. He has no dislikes or antipathies and hates no man except bigots and tyrants. He accepts knowledge although it comes from the humblest of sources; believes that there is no experience but that will repay a careful study of it. He believes that there is no husbandry's plowshare but that will turn up soil that is worth the analyzing. He belongs exclusively to no party, and he can be easily approached by respectable men of every stamp, whether belonging to the same party or school, or society with him or not. You can easily take hold of his nature and draw it out without having it slip from your fingers and fly back from your presence into a thousand kinks, just like an overtwisted string. He is a whole man. God made him for the whole world and not for a party. But by some strong influence you may draw him from the world for a time into some narrow sphere, but not only will his reluctant nature, like a returning tide, run back continuedly to embrace the continent, and, like a full sea, come back boiling and bubbling and running all over.

WHAT WE WANT.

In order that medical knowledge may increase its liberality in the true and full sense, we want true men in high places, who will not only let their own light shine everywhere, but will cease to hinder other men's light from shining. Beyond this, and of equal importance with it, we want the medical Pearls of Wisdom and Gems of Knowledge diffused among the people; we want what the world has never seen before—a popular medical literature. We want the Temple of Esculapius pulled down and these conservative priests turned into the street to become teachers of the multitude, rather than the worshippers of the inner sanctuary. We do not think it necessary to confine knowledge, save in the ministers of religion. Why should not the layman, who follows his plow or shoves the plane, become eminent theologians? And why should they not study the lower branches of science which relate to the body? They have never done it heretofore just because it has been purposely hidden from them under technicalities, when those covers should have been torn from them. And they will be in the very near future, for when men and women are educated properly, as they should be and must be, how the physical temple can be built, then taught how they should take care of it as well, then the soul will need but very little doctoring to save it. It is said those who begin to read upon medicine are very apt to imagine themselves afflicted with the various symptoms that they find described. Well, to some extent, they may. But it is also true that the light they obtain by reading very often relieves their minds of the apprehension which their previous ignorance allowed to prey upon them, just as boys lose their fears of ghosts, when the light of the coming morn changes their thoughts to some familiar object. But those conserva tive physicians oppose the spread of medical knowledge; they fear that their services will be less required—I fear upon the grounds of self interest. They think that their services will be less sought for.

Now, we do not think of dispensing with the clergy because the people study theology; neither do we cease to employ teachers and practitioners of medicine when each man and woman will study the healing art. The principal change we shall witness in the future will be much larger attainments in knowledge among practitioners, just as ministers now know, and are obliged to know, just ten times as much as they did know in the dark ages of the past, when the people had no education and were obliged to receive their spiritual teaching from the mouths of those old fossils. The teachers of any art or science are obliged to keep in advance of their pupils. Just let the study of medicine become a popular study among the people, and then we will have very few ignorant physicians as we do now. Quacks will then become one of the impossibilities. The eclectic and the homeopathic as well as all true physicians believe in scattering medical books among the people, stripped of their technicalities.

Diffuse the Pearls of Wisdom and the Gems of Knowledge, and you will find that the people will purchase very few of the secret advertised medicines, nor employ quacks as their family physicians.

Hygiene.

Hygiene differs from medicine, but bears a close relationship to it. Hygiene prevents disease, and medicine cures disease. Hygiene bears a close connection to physiology, which teaches the laws of life and health; to chemistry, which reveals the nature of poisons, whether taken in the air we breathe, the food we eat, or the fluids we drink. Hygiene aims to discover the cause of disease and death, and the means of averting or altering these causes so as to prevent these calamities. To do this it classifies the factors of life under AIR, FOOD, WATER, and HEAT.

There can be no animal life without AIR. The smallest insect needs a supply of oxygen gas. This it must draw from the atmosphere, and when once obtained, it produces its chemical changes in the interior of the insect. Each living cell of which its body is composed, contributes to the aggregate of its life, only as it is acted upon by the oxygen received. It is this fact that lies at the foundation of a thousand enquiries in regard to the ventilation of dwellings, workshops, churches, etc.; indeed, of all places where there are living beings. By this great fact we are enabled to explain a large per cent. of disease and death, and the more this is studied and heeded, the more will longevity be promoted, and the health of cities and communities enhanced. But we are also to remember, that the air we breathe not only supplies us with oxygen, but it is the great repository of all the exhalants from the earth and decayed animal and vegetable matter. It comes to us sometimes loaded with poisons. Being absorbed into the blood, they work their destructive action on the body, damaging the functions of life, and often destroying the existence altogether.

WATER is another factor of organic life. Without it, no chemical change can take place in the living body. Water enters into all the composition of organized beings. A man that weighs 150 pounds, contains 111 pounds of water in his tissues. All the solid materials of the body are carried to their places by the agency of water. All the higher animals drink water for this very purpose; and the adult human being takes, upon an average, from seventy to eighty ounces of water daily. Water is a most potent chemical agent; its solvent power is equal to that of the mineral acids, and it associates itself with a vast number of compounds. It dissolves both organic and inorganic matter; but it may become so impregnated with poisonous substances as to unfit it for the purposes of life.

But the human body requires varied compounds of carbon, hydrogen, oxygen and nitrogen in the shape of FOOD. Air and water, of themselves, though they fill an important place in the economy of life, cannot supply the system with elements necessary for the play of chemical forces which result in vital phenomena. The blood must be supplied with chloride and sulphate of lime, the muscles must have potash, the bile must have sulphur, the saliva cyanogen, the nerves phosphorus, the hair, teeth and nails must have silica. If the diet is deficient, disease will invade the system most certainly. Armies have been starved on an excessive diet of salt beef. Children have been sacrificed by a confinement to starchy food. The human body may have too much of one thing and not enough of another. What then is a healthy diet? We answer, such diet as contains the constituents o the human body. Science and instinct both answer this question. They reach the same goal, and, in this connection, comes up the question of nervous stimulants as tea, coffee, tobacco, opium and alcoholic drinks, for which we have no space in this little volume. Suffice it to say, they are not necessary except as medicines.

HEAT is one of the factors of life. Air, food, and water generate the heat of the body. Civilized man has instituted artificial heat, which, to a great degree, compensates for the lack of food. The savage and the animal may live without artificial heat by a ready supply of air, food and water. There is no life where the temperature never rises above 32 degrees F. A little above this, we find only plants and animals of the feeblest vitality. As we ascend the scale, we find animals and birds so constituted as to maintain their own temperature by supplies of food. If man's food is scant, he heaps on clothing; if his dwelling is warm, he requires less food and clothing.

Philosophy of Human Magnetism.

This is a very common superstition among popular medical men of all schools, that the intellectual phenomena of Magnetism (or Mesmerism) are the concomitants of hysterical states of the nervous system. Old-line doctors attempt to transcend the otherwise insurmountable difficulties of Somnambulism, or Clairvoyance, by the assumption of imposture, or else by charging the mental manifestation to nervous or cataleptic condition of body and brain. But, however, it is pretty generally believed that the majority of those old-line physicians are pretty well supplied with ignorance concerning many of the most vital processes of the physical organization. But chemistry has recently enriched the physicians' understanding of physiological phenomena, but chemistry does not unravel to his mind the wondrous dynamic of the feelings and thinking principles which animate and govern the perfect and beautiful organism of man and woman. The mental and spiritual phenomena of magnetism are yet new to most physicians, and, therefore, we do not expect anything else from them than expressions of professional prejudices emphasized by strong marks of dogmatic denunciations. But there is here and there a broad-hearted and knowledge-loving physician who is capable of putting a rational question with an honest incredulity, and who, consequently, is ever ready to exchange his learned errors for new truths—is willing to make progress in scientific facts, and thus unfurl the union banner of free thought and unlimited investigation. But in this little explanation it can hardly be expected of us to construct an argument for the establishment of electro-magnetic science; but we can scarcely believe that such an argument is demanded by the so-called scientists of the age, and yet we know that no class is more in the rear of advanced discovery than the graduates of our institutions of learning. Many of our best students in medicine are unable to solve the first group of magnetic phenomena. They treat the facts as obviously incredible and impossible, and so permit themselves to be sufficiently logical to reject the facts, and sometimes uncivil enough to insult the hewers of wood and drawers of water, who have the audacity to present such phenomena for scientific examination. In fact, the colleges and churches are both behind the essentials of knowledge and civilization. The unscientific people, the non-professional observers of nature, and the clear-eyed matronly nurse of the sick-room, are the unconscious champions of scientific progress.

After these, like a loaded omnibus behind the laboring horses, come the respectable hosts of physicians and clergymen riding and enjoying themselves luxuriously in the cushioned chairs of our colleges and evangelical institutions. Millions upon millions of human beings, as well as creatures of the lower grade of animation, breathe the breath of life all unconcious of science, unmindful of the chemical knowledge which would explain the composition of the atmosphere, and reveal the proportions of oxygen and nitrogen to the thoughtless multitude. So it is in every other respect. The people intuitively illustrate the essential facts of science for centuries in advance of the accurate knowledge of the schools. In *human magnetism*, this remark is emphatically true. The people with little or no education are familiar with its essential facts, and have practiced the principles of this science long eras before the colleges reflect a single ray of light upon the subject. In fact, the people, on the contrary, without education, are masters of realities and principles not yet dreamed of in the brains of our teachers and professors. For, in truth, what is science? Nothing more nor less than systematic observation and orderly arrangement of those natural facts and superficial causes which have for hundreds of centuries been common and familiar to some of the inhabitants of every country. It is, therefore, no disadvantage to any experience or philosphy to say that it is not yet accepted and inculcated by talented men in high places, because we know that the knowledge of the colleges and of the theology of the churches are but reflections of the facts and discoveries of the past ages.

WHAT IS THE SOURCE OF MAGNETISM?

Or, in other words, *what* is Magnetism? We answer, that it is animal vitality. We use the term Magnetism in its broadest sense, signifying the principle by which one object is enabled to attract, repel and influence another. The *source* of this grand principle is *Soul*. Crystals, various mineral bodies, plants, trees, fish, birds, animals, human beings, each and all are endowed with this magnetic principle, because each and all are endowed with a soul, which is the mystic life of all boundless nature upwelling and overflowing from the inexhaustible fountain of the First Cause. All students who are intellectually acquainted with the harmonial philosophy will not confound " Soul and Spirit." The term "Soul" is used here to signify that harmonious combination of the principle of motion, life, and sensation, which moves, warms and perfects the physical organizations. Stones, trees, animals and men all contain this principle, but the latter in a higher degree of development, while in the former the principle is comparatively dormant. Each natural body of matter is differently capacitated; hence, also, is it differently supplied with a soul principle. The consequence of this difference is a magnetic polarity between one body and another throughout the entire domain of nature, and the consequence of this universal polarity is evolution and manifestation of all the physical motions and mental phenomena known or unknown to science.

FACTS ILLUSTRATIVE OF MAGNETIC POLARITY.

The common magnet, as every one knows, is at once positive and negative; that is, the life of the metallic body makes two manifestations at the same moment, and will attract a negative substance and repel that which is positive to it. The positive pole is charged with negative power, and the negative pole with positive power. Thus the magnetic principle corresponds to these facts. For instance, the seed of a plant is negative to the magnetic ray or heat of the sun; consequently, the properties of the seed, if planted in good ground, leap up toward the sun as naturally as the needle points to the pole. This explains the growth of vegetables. Thus the near relationship of magnetism and electricity is demonstrated; they mutually attract and mutually repel each other. Look at the common electro-magnetic battery. If the electric current is permitted to traverse the coil of wire, it will convert the rod of iron placed in the center into a powerful magnet, and thus it in its turn will set in motion a powerful current of electricity, as it were, by way of compensation.

Now, the human body is constituted on the same system of polarities. Man is polarized from side to side, from end to end, from center to surface; his nervous system is a net-work of polarities, from his inmost organic centers to the glands of his brain, and from his brain centers to the extremities of every nerve; he is a perfect battery of magnetic and electric potence. Hence, you can see how easy it is to understand how individuals can affect each other magnetically, and assist in establishing a healthy equilibrium in the magnetical polarities of the human system; for the entire left side from the brain to the toes is negative; the left side emanations are, therefore, tranquil and attractive, while in the right side, which is positive, the emanations are powerfully repellant. Hence, man repels and works and destroys with his right side, right arm, right hand, right leg, right foot and brain, while with the corresponding parts and members of the left side and brain he attracts and subdues, and magnetizes whatever he is adapted to affect.

The right side of the brain is frequently unimpressible, while the left side may be easily overcome and paralyzed by the magnetic principle of another mind. The right eye in a healthy person is the keenest and best, while the left eye is capable of more pleasureable visions. The left eye is more susceptible for this reason: it more readily discerns the colors of a substance. The location, the size, the weight, and the distance of a body are quicker determined by the right eye. If any of you doubt this, go and experiment with your eyes and senses. Close your left eye and look at the leaf of a plant, then reverse the method, and you will soon begin to see the ray of light emanating from the leaf which your right eye cannot discover.

In like mannar your left hand will detect heat in a substance that is cold to the right hand, and the reverse is equally true when frequently practiced with care and discrimination. For these reasons the right hand of man and woman are attractive to each other, while, at the same time the hand of the same sex are mutually repellant and unwholesome. Now clairvoyants can detect the emanations of the different centers by the colors, which is natural to all polarized principles. Clairvoyants can see the magnetic emanations from human bodies when they are in this illuminated state, and such sensitive persons are often repelled away from gross positive minds, and shun them as we would shun a viper, and our professors of science call such delicate natures weak-minded persons, when the fact is just the reverse·

Such minds as those always have far more intellectual brain power than the former.

The wonderful complex nervous system of man is a complete helix; a coil of wire which communicates electricity to the brain, which is the magnet, or central power of the organization, and the compensating process as with the electro-battery goes on in the shape of centrifugal currents of real nerve life, (a finer electricity), which the brain discharges through the pneumogastric sympathetic nerves to all parts of the temple. So, in accord with the magnetic law, we come now to observe that the brain and body of the operator becomes one overmastering, positive power, to which, without resistance, the diseased patient surrenders to the positive healthy magnetism of the operator. Thus the complete blending of the magnetic spheres of the twain, the disease in the patient naturally surrenders itself to the healthy body of the operator. Thus, you see, it is only a question of time, either long or short, which must, of necessity, equalize the magnetic soul principle, and both become healthy alike. This magnetic law lies at the foundation of all the so-called Spiritual Phenomena, wherein, to the observer, it seems that the spirit or mind of the medium has vacated its temple in order to give a foreign intelligence an opportunity of manifesting itself.

MAGNETISM AS A MEDICINE.

Having briefly sketched the action and effects of the magnetic principles, it will now be more expedient to conclude our remarks in behalf of the sick and suffering. The human body, in its normal and healthy condition, is endowed with every requisite power. But by ignorant and negligent treatment the natural vital forces lose their just equilibrium, and the effects and consequences are soon visible in material prostration, in severe pain, or in silent and insensible decomposition. What physicians term "nervous influence" is really nothing but the magnetic and electric life of the interior soul. Animals, including man, have these magnetic endowments; and the principle of vital action, in both the human and animal kingdom are exactly and universally identical. A loss of vital action is nothing but a loss of balance between inherent forces, which are positive and negative, or magnetic or electric; and yet we do not hold that the currents generated by the *metalic*, or mineral battery can ever be made to act as a substitute, because the principles of *Soul-Life* are as much finer than atmospheric electricity as the latter is finer and more delicate than the gross and turbulent waters of our lakes.

The Therepeutic influence of magnetism may be exerted in various ways, differing, in every case, with temperaments and the nature of the disease; but we cannot stop now to specify any methods. We will say, however, that it must be borne in mind that to practice Magnetic Healing successfully, you must have an *active will* to do *good;* a firm faith in your power, and an active confidence in employing it. Magnetism is a useful, a spiritualizing, and a sublime agent of vital energy and health. In fact, it is the all-pervading sympathy which connects us with the absolute condition and suffering of our fellowmen. However, we prescribe different remedies merely as palliatives and aids as final redemption from disease, and from the fear of death, but the radical remedy is still within your own individual organization. We have now given you the general principles of the magnetic medicine treasured up in the organs and brain-centers of your own individuality, An inflammation is a positive condition of an organ or part; therefore, apply your positive hand and *will* to it. Why? Because two positives repel, and your hand being a healthy positive, will surely scatter the inflammation, which is an unhealthy positive, and thus establish the natural equilibrium. Your brain, for instance, is loaded with blood; not so, your mental magnet is surcharged and overstocked with vital currents which should be engaged in other parts of your economy—and thus the dependent blood is floated off. So our doctors will bleed an apoplectic patient. This method is absurd. No man's system ever generates more blood than it needs for its own private use. But it is possible, nay, easy for the magnetic potencies to be thrown out of balance, giving rise to co-ordinate symptoms of excess in one place, and of deficiency in another; the remedy, in all cases, being the same, viz: A restoration of the magnetic equilibrium between foot and brain, between stomach and liver, between heart and lungs, between spleen and kidneys, and the inevitable consequences will be perfect health.

Dr. H. S. Tanner's Fast.

Just as we are finishing our last manuscript for our book, Dr. H. S. Tanner has at last completed his forty days without food, and thirteen of which were passed without drink.

Having been criticized for honest assertion of a former fast of forty-two days, by Dr. Hammond, of New York, and others of like belief and persuasion, the Doctor took up a temporary residence in New York City, under the charge of the United States Medical College, for the purpose of convincing the most skeptical of the entire possibility of a man existing forty days without food.

Notwithstanding the Doctor had to brave all former theorizers and the bulwark of "old hunker medicine," he most assiduously pursued his attempt, under the most trying ordeal and adverse circumstances, to a successful termination, and on Saturday, August 7, 1880, he completed such an abstinence as never before has been authoritatively recorded—notwithstanding Dr. Hammond and Dr. Clendenin, Health Officer Dr. Miles, and many others of the most brilliant shining stars of the Allopathic School said that it could not be done, and pronounced Dr. Tanner a humbug and a fraud.

But long before Dr. Tanner had completed his forty days' fast in New York, the public generally was satisfied that he was honestly attempting to carry out what he had undertaken. And those of the profession who at first claimed that a fast of forty days was impossible, gradually began to change front, and to affirm that such facts were not new, and that many well authenticated cases were on record, and that they had proved of no benefit to science. After which came the prediction of the knowing ones, that Dr. Tanner would suffer greatly and probably die as soon as he began to take nourishment, for such had been the result of all cases of starvation, and Dr. Tanner could not be an exception to the general rule.

That fasts of this kind were possible, Dr. Tanner always held, and one of his objects in undertaking so trying an ordeal was to prove that such things could be done. Many cases of fasting had been reported, but they were rarely believed, for the reason that no positive evidence of such fasting could be furnished, except such as was given by the faster. Dr. Tanner, however, accomplished his task under the most rigid system of scrutiny, and the eyes of the whole world upon him. Thus giving positive proof of the possibility of a protracted fasting. Therefore, when we have demonstrated to us that medical authorities are in error regarding the length of time life may be prolonged without food, we are brought face to face with some of the errors we are guilty of in our daily visits to patients, it matters little what the disease may be; we have been disposed to urge the taking of food to sustain life, even if our patient protested against it. This has especially been the custom of the profession during the last decade, since the supporting and nourishing system of practice came into use. But now it has become a question whether food thus taken when the system did not demand it, had any effect in sustaining life, and whether nature is not the best guide after all as to the necessity for food being taken into the stomach.

And now, that it is demonstrated that a person can go ten, twenty or even forty days without food, then it is plainly our duty to cure the disease by cutting short the irritation by forcing food upon the stomach when it does not require it. If we have an inflamed eye, we give it rest, and it is rapidly restored. Therefore, the same treatment adopted for diseases of the digestive organs must necessarily be followed by equally good results; and Dr. Tanner has taught the world that we can abstain from food for comparatively long periods of time without bad results.

Again, the leading authorities have taught us that after long abstinence from food the digestive organs are so impaired that food must be given in very minute quantities. This practice is adopted in all cases of starvation, and it is a fact that nearly all such patients die. Now Dr. Tanner has shown that long abstinence does not impair digestion, but that large quantities of nourishment can be taken with impunity. Therefore, a change in this direction promises good results, and should be considered one of the lessons of the fast.

This fast farther demonstrates that even rectal feeding does not sustain life, as has been claimed; but rather that the other forces of the body not only keep the patient alive, but also counteract the bad effects of this false method of supposed feeding.

The most important fact proven by this fast is the wonderful power of mind over matter, as we have tried to explain to you (see article on Human Magnetism). This fact has demonstrated to science clearly that the human mind is dependent upon some force outside of the physical brain. Thus, to our mind, it has only added another link to the chain of evidence which we already have, that the mind or spirit, or whatever you wish to call it, does control the body and does live after the body is all used up and worn out and laid away to mingle with the rubbish of the graveyard.

In fact, there are so many points which present themselves for our consideration in this great lesson of the Dr. Tanner fast and feast, that we can do little at present but turn the facts to practical use, and mark out a course for future study, since after the fast came the feast, when it seems that Dr. Tanner knew the powers of his stomach better than the medical savants, and at once began to partake of large quantities of food from a generous bill of fare, and in four days he gained twenty-four pounds in weight; and now, the 31st day of August, just twenty-six days since he completed his fast, he has regained his usual weight and strength, and is as well and hearty as ever.

INDEX.

	PAGE.
A GOOD NURSE	7
Kind of nurses	9
The lazy nurse	10
The cruel nurse	10
The careless nurse	10
The fussy nurse	10
The dishonest nurse	11
The tattling nurse	11
ACCIDENTS AND EMERGENCIES	50
Burns and scalds	50
Poison vine; poison oak	51
Spider bites	52
Snake bites	52
Cramp in stomach	52
Bilious colic or cramp colic	53
Jaundice	53
Neuralgia	54
Earache	54
Diphtheria	55
Erysipelas	56
Scarlet fever	58
Small pox	59
Worms	60
Chronic sore eyes	61
Sick headache	62
Chronic rheumatism	63
Sunstroke	65
Cholera morbus	66
Cholera infantum	67
Measles	68
Catarrh	69
Gonorrhea	71
Diabetes	73
Asthma	74
Pneumonia	76
Gravel	77
Spermatorrhea	80
Suppression of monthly periods	83
Dymenorrhea	83
Menorrhagia	84
Cessation of the menses	85
St. Vitus' dance	86

	PAGE.
Catalepsy	86
Epilepsy	87
Paralysis	88
Dyspepsia	89
Dropsy	91
Intermittent fever	92
BATH	28
The foot bath	29
The hip, or sitz bath	30
CAUSE AND CURE OF FEMALE WEAKNESS	46
DR. JONES' HOME TURKISH BATH	93
DR. TANNER'S FAST	144
EATING	22
FEVERS	30
Rules to observe	31
FOOD AND DRINK FOR THE SICK	13
GENERAL REMARKS	121
HEMORRHAGE	33
Bleeding and how to stop it	33
Bleeding from nose	34
Bleeding above the ear	34
Bleeding below the eyes	34
Bleeding from a wound in arm	34
Bleeding from a wound in leg or foot	35
Bleeding from the stomach	35
Bleeding from the lungs	35
HISTORY AND ORIGIN OF MEDICINE	122
Present medical schools	124
Progress of medicine	131
Need of liberality	132
Medical science	133
Conservative leaders	133
The true physician	134
What we want	135
HYGIENE	136
INFECTIOUS DISEASES	37
Whooping cough	38
Croup	38
Children's convulsions or fits	39
Diarrhea	40
Dysentery or bloody flux	41
LUNG LIFE	23
MEDICINES FOR A HAPPY HOME	42
MOTHERHOOD	43
MAXIMS	45
PHILOSOPHY OF HUMAN MAGNETISM	138
What is the source of magnetism?	140
Facts illustrative of magnetic polarity	140
Magnetism as a medicine	142
POISON AND THEIR ANTIDOTES	115
Arsenic	116
Copper	116
Iron	116

INDEX.

	PAGE.
Lead	117
Phosphorus	117
Opium	117
Strychnine	117
Other poisonous plants or seeds	118
RECIPES FOR COOKING	**14**
Beef tea	14
Extract of beef	14
Chicken jelly	14
Barley water	15
Rice water	15
Arrowroot jelly	15
Barley jelly	15
Oat meal gruel	15
Corn meal gruel	16
Oat meal water	16
Buttermilk pap	16
Wine whey	16
Orange whey	16
Vegetable soup	17
Elm-bark jelly	17
Flax-seed lemonade or cough syrup	17
Milk punch	17
RECIPES, ETC.	**95**
Constipation of the bowels	95
Common bilious condition	96
Cholera infantum	96
Catarrh of the bladder	97
Malarial affections	97
Rheumatism	97
How to prevent a felon	98
Bone felons, carbuncles and boils	98
Poison oak or ivy	98
Chapped hands, face or lips	99
Convulsions in little children	99
Summer diarrhea in children	99
Rickety children	99
Rheumatic gout	100
Profuse menstruation	100
Painful Menstruation	100
Excess of vomiting	101
Nipple wash	101
Nursing sore mouth	101
Tonic for disease of the kidney	102
Inaction of the kidneys	102
Diptheria	102
Erysipelas	103
Rheumatism	103
Dressing for burns and ulcers	104
Earache	104
For the itch	104
Lost appetite	104
Magnetic liniment for rheumatism, sprains or stiff joints	105

	PAGE.
Magnetic lotion for the human body	105
Dr. Jones' restorative compound	106
Catarrh snuff	107
Powders for cramp in the stomach, or diophoretic powder	107
Dysentery—bloody flux	108
Piles—Hemorrhoids	108
Cough syrups	109
Sprains	110
Healing salve	110
Cure for bunions or frost-bitten feet	111
Scurvy	111
Miscellaneous	111
Ringworm and tetter	112
Enlargement of the spleen	112
For the kidneys in dropsical affections	112
How to prepare poultices	112
How to make fomentations	114
Valuable tooth wash	115
Toooth-ache	115
RULES TO ADMINISTER MEDICINE	119
To measure medicine, instead of weighing	119
Liquid measure	120
Dry measure	120
Doses of Medicine	120
SINGULAR PHYSIOLOGICAL FACTS	24
Process of digestion	25
The purifying ordeal of the blood	25
Remedy for constipation	26
Neuralgia	27
THE ROOM FOR THE SICK	12
THE LITTLE INFANT	18
Teething	20
THE HOME MEDICINE CHEST	32
WOUNDS	36
Broken bones and dislocations	36

www.ingramcontent.com/pod-product-compliance
Lightning Source LLC
Chambersburg PA
CBHW030345170426
43202CB00010B/1254